The Hea

Black Cumin

Sylvia Luetjohann

The Healing Power
of
Black Cumin

A Handbook on Oriental Black Cumin Oils
Their Healing Components and Special Recipes

Translated by Christine M. Grimm

LOTUS LIGHT
SHANGRI-LA

1st English edition 1998
© by Lotus Light Publications
    Box 325, Twin Lakes, WI 53181
The Shangri-La Series is published in cooperation
with Schneelöwe Verlagsberatung, Federal Republic of Germany
© 1997 reserved by the Windpferd Verlagsgesellschaft mbH, Aitrang
All rights reserved
Translated by Christine M. Grimm
Cover design by Kuhn Grafik, Digitales Design, Zurich, illustration by
Elisabeth Pabst
Illustrations: Elisabeth Pabst
Photographs: p. 16 – Lavendelfoto/Beat Ernst,
p. 44 – Dr. Refai, p. 45, 46 und 47 – Renate Spannagel
Composition and make-up: *panta rhei!* – MediaService Uwe Hiltmann
Production: Schneelöwe, D-87648 Aitrang

ISBN 0-914955-53-5
Library of Congress Catalogue No. 97-76440

Printed in the USA

Table of Contents

THE AREAS OF APPLICATION

A Preface of Thanks

As I set out on the sometimes difficult and confusing search for clues about black cumin, which is quite versatile in every respect, a lucky coincidence had me meet Dr. Diab Refai, a doctor of Syrian origin. Thanks to him, much first-hand information about Arabian traditions, therapeutic applications, and quality characteristics could flow into this book. His enthusiasm and personal dedication provided decisive inspiration for the work.

In addition, I would like to thank Elisabeth Pabst who, with her profuse botanic knowledge and illustrations reflecting the spirit of the plant, has also contributed much to the successful completion of this book; "Nigellina," Renate Spannagel for her warmhearted and accomplished commitment not only in Turkey; and my publisher, Monika Jünemann, who was not only substantially involved in nurturing the work but also lent practically untiring outer support and helped calm down the inner surges.

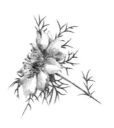

Introduction

Black Cumin—A Rediscovered Miracle Cure?

In the Mediterranean countries and the Near East, black cumin has already been considered a medicinal plant and the oil from its seeds a "miracle cure" for thousands of years. The saying handed down from the Prophet Mohammed: "Black cumin heals every disease—except death" has certainly made a significant contribution to black cumin's living tradition in most Islamic nations. Even today, it has a high standing as the "medicine of the Prophet" that is extremely versatile in its application.

In earlier days, black cumin was also very valued in the Central European latitudes as a medicinal and spice plant, but for many years now only the variety with the botanic name of *Nigella damascena* has adorned our country gardens as the particularly attractive "love-in-a-mist."

In recent times, however, black cumin has also been rediscovered here as a medicinal plant, and modern research is now looking for scientific proof for the qualities that have been attributed to the realm of the purely empirical art of healing. This means: modern medical and biochemical research methods have been used for the past few years to get to the bottom of the experiences of the ancient Assyrians and Egyptians skilled in the art of healing.

Since black cumin—as also many comparable medicinal plants—is a distinctly complex remedy with more than one-hundred components working together synergetically, the research is far from complete. We still don't have exact information about 6% of the ingredients of the valuable oil pressed from the seeds, and these in particular could be highly effective. Nevertheless, it can be said that the results of the studies up to now in the USA and Europe have already surpassed expectations. This applies especially to the effect

11

of black cumin oil on the immune system and therefore to areas like allergies, which are otherwise considered to be therapy-resistant. People with allergies require an increased supply of polyunsaturated fatty acids, which are contained at a high concentration in black cumin oil. With these as basic building blocks, certain tissue hormones (prostaglandins) are formed within the organism. These not only have an anti-inflammatory and bronchodilatory effect but also have a regulating and harmonizing influence on the immune system. In addition, lowered physical resistance is not only the cause of increased susceptibility to infections: almost all people suffering from chronic diseases are affected by a weakened immune system.

Because of harmful environmental influences and metabolic disturbances on the basis of an improper diet, our immune resistance is at the mercy of intensive stress and faced with great challenges. As a food supplement, black cumin oil can offer valuable services here—in a natural way, without side effects or intolerance with another type of medical treatment. Yet, this far from exhausts its range of effectiveness: digestion disorders and kidney stones, the premenstrual syndrome, and menopausal complaints, sleep disturbances and weak concentration can be named as examples of the many application possibilities that have brought black cumin its almost legendary reputation as an ancient Oriental "miracle cure."

This book quite consciously follows the basic idea of capturing as much information as is possible and available at the current time and passing it on to the reader. It therefore ranges from old folk tradition and healing knowledge that has been handed down through generations, up to the latest medical findings and gas-chromatographic analyses and cosmetic and culinary recipes—a range that this "plant for our age" appears to sustain quite well…. Decide for yourself whether this externally rather modest plant represents the rediscovery of a medicinal plant that deserves your attention. You can become acquainted with it in the excursions through history and botany, illustrated by old recipes from various traditions of folk medicine, through modern research findings and advanced developments related to the current level of knowledge, complemented by personal experiences and case histories.

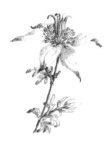

INTERESTING FACTS FROM THE LONG TRADITION OF AN ANCIENT MEDICINAL AND SPICE PLANT

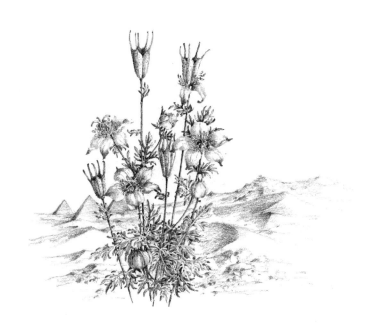

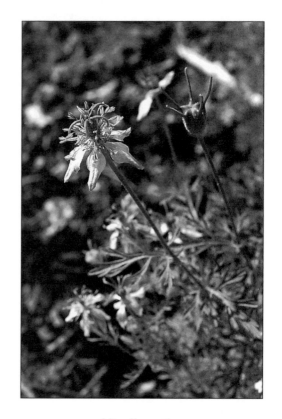

Nigella sativa

The Oriental Roots

Black cumin, a plant from the family of the crowfoot (ranunculus) plants, originates in the Mediterranean region and is indigenous to the countries of North Africa, the Near East, and Southeastern Europe. The earliest cultivation and use can be traced back more than 3,000 years to the kingdom of the Assyrians and ancient Egypt.

In an Assyrian herbal book, black cumin or "black tin-tir" is mentioned as a remedy that already had a variety of applications attributed to it: internally for the stomach, externally for treatment of the eyes, ears, and mouth, as well as for a great many skin problems like itching, rashes, sores, and herpes. Later, Pliny recommended that a mixture of crushed black cumin seeds, vinegar, and honey be smeared into a wound for first aid in the case of snake bite or scorpion sting, which has already been tested since time immemorial.

From the realm of the Pharaohs, tradition has it that black cumin was used as a digestive after opulent feasts, as well as a remedy for inflammations and certain hypersensitive reactions of the body that we today call "allergies." Proof of effectiveness for specific substances in inflammatory and allergic processes has already been provided by modern research results. Moreover, the legendary "bronze complexion" of the ancient Egyptians is attributed to the skin-care properties of black cumin oil. It is quite likely that these were also known to Queen Nofretete, who was praised for her beauty 1,350 years before our era. A great deal of speculation has already taken place about the discovery of a little bottle of black cumin oil in the tomb chamber of Tut-enkhamun—which is fitting for a miracle plant. It was even raised to the position of a companion for the life in the afterworld, although it obviously was incapable of preventing death. Perhaps this oil was simply considered to be a precious object for inclusion in the grave?

The Copts, as the Christian descendants of the ancient Egyptians, made sure that the tradition of herbal medicine remained alive. They also passed their knowledge on to the other peoples of the Arabian world. In Arabic, black cumin is called *kamûn asvad*, and High Arabic has the word *shouniz* for it as well; in addition, it also bears the names *habbe sôda*, "black seed," or *habbe el-barake*, the "inexhaustibly rich seed." The last term is derived from the Prophet Mohammed's praise already mentioned at the beginning: "Black cumin heals every disease—except death," which was recorded in the *Hadith "El Buchari."* Without a doubt, this quote has contributed to the great propagation of black cumin in the Islamic nations.

At the beginning of the 11th century, black cumin was mentioned extensively by the famous Persian doctor and philosopher Ibn Sina (also known as *Avicenna*) in his eminent medical treatise *Kitabasch schifa* (Book of Recovery) as having the following effects:

- Inner purification and detoxification of the body
- Reduction of mucous and strengthening of the lungs
- Home remedy against fever, coughs, colds, toothache and headache
- Remedy against skin diseases and for treatment of wounds
- Remedy against intestinal parasites and worms, as well as against bites and stings by poisonous animals.

The tradition in the Orient, which has been substantiated by many recipes, asserts its effects for gastrointestinal complaints, flatulence, diarrhea and constipation, jaundice and gallstones, for the stimulation of the kidneys and increased urination, against infections, congestion, and bronchial disorders, in case of menstrual complaints and for the promotion of lactation, against skin parasites, and as a vermicide especially for children. It also has been traditionally used by the people for skin-care and as a hair-care remedy against dandruff and hair loss. Even today, it can be found everywhere in the Oriental spice bazaars. The Turkish name *çöre-*

kotu, which can be approximately translated as "grass for little pastry," indicates a further way of putting it to use. Similar to poppy seed or sesame, it is sprinkled on flat breads. Many Muslims take a pinch of the seed in honey to strengthen their virility, among other things.

In Turkey there is also the tradition of using it as an incense, as well as the folk practice of sewing exactly 41 seeds of the black cumin into colorful little cloth sacks and then attaching them with a safety pin to the children's clothing. This talisman is meant to protect them. The seeds are also strung like pearls on strings and, decorated with colorful rags, hung in the window. Such a *nazarlik* is thought to protect people against the "evil eye."

From Southeastern Europe (Greece and Bulgaria) and North Africa (Sudan, Ethiopia, Egypt) through the Near Eastern countries of the Mediterranean, Syria, Turkey, ancient Mesopotamia, Persia, and Pakistan, black cumin reached India and even China. In India, black cumin is primarily cultivated in the regions of Punjab, Himachal Pradesh, Bihar, and Assam. Used as a medicine, *kalonji*, the "black onion seed," was and is still considered to be a tasty spice for supporting the metabolism, as well as a remedy for digestive disorders and the feared diarrhea diseases like amebic dysentery and shigellosis. In addition to the seeds and the fatty oil, essential black cumin oil also has a long tradition of use.

According to the Ayurvedic tradition and the typology of the three *doshas*, black cumin reduces *vata* and *kapha* and increases *pitta*. As a result, treatments even have been developed for such unusual indications as anorexia, certain disorders of the nervous system, discharge and venereal disease. Furthermore, gynecology plays a special role since black cumin—as a result of its uterus-contracting effect—is also administered when labor is weak and in cases of sepsis. However, because of the possibility of premature birth or miscarriage, should not be taken during pregnancy. In addition, a generally stimulating, tonicising, and mood-brightening effect is attributed to the seeds.

A common custom in all of India is to scatter the crushed *kalonji* seeds between clothes and scarves as an insect repellent. The anti-bacterial effect of the seeds is also well-known, making them suitable for the preservation of food as well.

The European Tradition—Part I

Black cumin is not only mentioned in *The Bible*, where it has the name *ketzah*, as a spice for bread and cake that can be used in a variety of ways, but was also known to all the naturopathic authors of Greek and Roman antiquity. The Greek physician Hippocrates (5th century B.C.) used the names *melánthion* (black leaf) or *meláspermon* (black seed) for it. The black seeds have also given the plant its botanical name, *Nigella* (from Latin *niger* = black or *nigellus* = blackish). In the first century of our age, it was treated extensively by Pliny the Elder in his extensive *Naturalis historia* (Natural History). The name appears here as *git* or *gith*, a term often used in ancient Latin writings that was probably derived from the Arabic language and which we will also encounter again frequently in the old German sources. An apparently also Arabicized form of black cumin's name—*salusandriam*—was used just a short time later than Pliny by the Greek physician Dioscurides in his five-volume pharmacology *De materia medica,* which was to influence the art of healing with plants far beyond the time of the Middle Ages.

Pliny lists a series of therapeutic applications, many of which we are already familiar with from the Arabian world, which naturally include the digestant effect as a bread seasoning; furthermore, the treatment of snake bites and scorpion stings that has already been mentioned, as well as callosities, old tumors, abscesses, skin rashes, and even freckles. An entire series of recipes with black cumin against colds and inflammations in the area of the head are recommended, and these appeared in an almost unchanged form many centuries later in the large German medicinal plant encyclopedias of the 16th to 18th centuries. Here are some samples from the *Naturalis Historia*:

> *Crushed and tied into a little linen cloth for the purpose of smelling, it drives away rhinitis (runny nose); spread with vinegar against headaches; spread into the nose with iris oil, catarrh of the conjunctiva and tumors; boiled with vinegar, toothaches; ground and chewed, ulcers in the mouth; drunk with the addition of sodium carbonate, breathing difficulties...*

The use of black cumin as a delicious and simultaneously curative bread seasoning was apparently able to assert itself in the following period of time in Germany. Around the year 794, its cultivation was recommended in the *Capitulare de villis* by Charlemagne for this intended purpose. Here it is often given the name of "Roman cumin" or "black coriander" and also had attributed to it the Arabian curative effects and those that had been handed down by Pliny. In the year 816, black cumin was listed in the "Hortus" of the St. Gallen monastery's map under the name of *gitto*. In Old German commentaries, it was called *protvurz* or *brotchrut*. The adaptation of the botanic name *Nigella* in the Middle Ages appears to primarily have its origins in the writings of Albertus Magnus, as well as establishing itself in pharmacology.

However, St. Hildegard of Bingen, who wrote her famous double work on biology and the art of healing in the 12th century, appears to regard black cumin with some suspicion. Although she very aptly assesses it to be a "plant of warm and dry quality," she then treats it in a strikingly brusque manner. Above all, the use of crushed black cumin seeds with fried bacon as a healing ointment against head ulcers is mentioned. The seed, mixed with honey and spread on the wall, is also recommended as a surefire flycatcher! However, with respect to consumption by human beings, St. Hildegard warns about its possibly toxic effect. This is definitely applicable to certain members of this rather branched crowfoot family. But since St. Hildegard gives the field black cumin the botanic name of *Githerum ratde* in her *Physica*, it is highly probably that the later notorious confusion with the corn cockle (*Agrostémma githago*) took place here. The seeds of this grain weed, feared by farmers, are actually poisonous because of saponins. They not only make flour, bread, and grain coffee bitter, but are also even harmful to health.

Despite this, the reputation of black cumin as a healing remedy must have stabilized itself in folk medicine during the course of the next centuries and even continued to spread since a considerable abundance of knowledge about *Nigella*, now also generally called "black coriander," was demonstrated in the publication of the *New Kreutterbuch* by Hieronymus Bock in 1539. At latest at this point, the path of our search for traces appears to be blocked by a rank growth of different plants, often difficult to penetrate, with deviating descriptions and increasingly imaginative names. This appears to make a side-trip into the world of botany necessary.

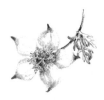

Botanical and Other Excursions Through the Most Important Species of Black Cumin

Black cumin is an annual plant that is propagated by sowing or propagates itself. However, despite the name and partially similar uses, there is no botanical relationship to our spice caraway. Despite frequent confusion of the two, this also applies to the Indian cumin with its species of *Cuminum cyminum* and *Cuminum nigrum*. In contrast to these, black cumin does not belong to the umbelliters but rather to the crowfoot plants (ranunculaceae), which, in accordance with current findings, represent one of the plant families richest in alkaloids. The subgroup of the black cumin species distinguishes itself in particular because the five carpellary leaves that usually are located separated next to each other are more or less adnoted with each other in the middle in accordance with the particular species. This creates a wheel-shaped seed capsule or the so-called collective follicular fruit, the valves of which only separate in the middle when they are ripe. While the adnascence only goes halfway up in the less conspicuous wild sorts, the two best-known species, the true black cumin and the damascena black cumin have it all the way up to the tip so that the five pistils protruding beyond the perimeter of the wheel form the figure of a spiked wheel.

This has earned the plant the name of Catherine wheel since St. Catherine in the iconographic pictures is always portrayed with a spiked wheel. According to the legend, the wheel with which she was to suffer a martyr's death in the year 309 broke and she had to be executed with the sword. This is why she also just holds a fragment of a wheel in her hand in the pictures of her as a saint. Analogous to this, the Catherine wheel breaks into five parts when it is ripe and lets the seeds that have grown in two rows along the inner suture fall out.

Before we stray even further into the borderland between folkloristic botany and legends, the three most important species of black cumin should now be described.

Nigella sativa, the true or common black cumin, is a plant with a height of 30 to 50 centimeters and filigree appearance. It has an upright stem with few branches that is somewhat hirsute. The leaves are bipinnatified or tripinnatified, giving them a similarity to umbellifers like caraway, fennel, and coriander reflected in such forms of names like "Roman cumin," "fennel-flower," and "black coriander." From the individual apical blossoms, which are milky white and take on a bluish-greenish coloration close to the tip, the coarse pustule-covered, ball-like fruit capsules develop after the bloom. These are crowned by five protruding spikes reminiscent of beaks.

The black seeds of the nigella (*nigellus* = "blackish") are triangular and horizontally wrinkled, looking very much like onion seeds. The similarity of the fruit capsule with the poppy plant probably contributed to the botanical name *Papaver nigrum* or "black poppy," and in earlier times the seeds were even mixed with those of the thorn apple (datura), which is commonly called "black cumin."

Only the seeds and the oil pressed out of them are seen as medicinally significant components of the plant; this valuation is also reflected in the old name of "nard seeds," for example. When ground, they smell very aromatic—however, not like caraway but more like fennel or anise and are also reminiscent of nutmeg. This has inspired the names "fennel-flower" and "nutmeg-flower." The smell also sometimes conjures up associations with camphor or even cajaput. In terms of the taste, the seeds are piquant, slightly bitter, and have a pleasant spiciness to them so that people in earlier times liked to use them in place of common caraway, and they have even served as a pepper substitute. In France, *poivrette* (which can be translated something like "little pepper") is therefore the name of the Arabian spice *abésodé* that is crushed to make a powder.

Through extraction, as well as cold-pressing, the fatty oil with its valuable ingredients can be won from the seeds, whcih contain approx. 35% – 40% of the oil. Black cumin oil is said to have a more concentrated effect than the unproc-

The Most Important Species of Black Cumin

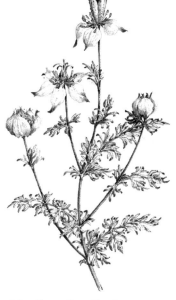

Nigella sativa, the true black cumin

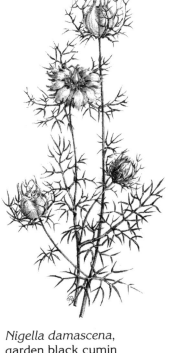

Nigella damascena, garden black cumin

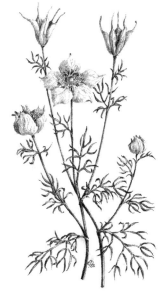

Nigella arvensis, field black cumin

essed seeds. By way of distillation, essential oil can also be extracted from the seeds and makes up approx. 0.5% – 1.5% of *Nigella sativa*. It has a yellowish to brownish color with a somewhat acrid smell and also has the characteristic of not being fluorescent.

At least twenty different varieties and crossbreeds of the black cumin are prevalent in the coastal countries of the Mediterranean and in the bordering regions, including both the wild and the cultivated species such as *Nigella aristata* and *Nigella orientalis*. The latter distinguishes itself by its strikingly light-green leaves and red-speckled yellow flowers, as well as the yellowish seeds. In general, the various nigella species can differ quite extensively from each other: the Syrian black cumin has quite large, light-blue flowers and longer, finer leaves in comparison to the Egyptian. This takes us to the next relative of the *Nigella sativa*—the *Nigella damascena*.

Nigella damascena, called Damask fennel (or Turkish black cumin) and also known as garden black cumin, is indigenous to the Mediterranean countries and the Near East as well. The name it has been given refers particularly to Turkey and Syria with its capital of Damascus. This species of nigella has become a favorite ornamental garden plant in Europe since about the middle of the 16th century. Because of its attractiveness, it enjoys greater popularity than the *Nigella sativa*, a fact supported by descriptions found in the old herbal books; not only was it illustrated more frequently than the latter but described to be "lovelier and more cheerful" because of the sky-blue of its rose-like flowers and the striking abundance of its little leaves that appeared to be as fine as hair. Above all, it awakened the associations with delicate girls, which is why it has received so many poetic names in folk botany and is surrounded by myths and legends.

The Damask fennel grows to be 75 centimeters tall and has an upright stem with dark-green, very finely slit leaves with long tips. These are not only reminiscent of dill leaves but also of a delicate wickerwork of roots or hair. In addition, the blossoms are surrounded by a so-called involucrum, a bracht hull of five similarly slit leaves. Their similarity to a spider has led this plant to be called "spider flower" in Switzerland. The sepals have a milky-white base but turn to a pale-blue color closer to the tip. At first glance, they could be taken to be flower petals, yet their somewhat coarsely veined structure and the coloring that tends towards green lets them be recognized as sepals.

The *Nigella damascena* primarily owes many of its very feminine names to its fine foliage, which permits conclusions about its sensitive nature. This garden plant is usually known as "love in a mist," a name is related to the myth about the German Emperor Frederick I's death by drowning during a campaign in Asia Minor:

On an expedition to the Holy Land, Emperor Frederick I Barbarossa built his camp on the shore of the Kalikaduus River. He went for a walk there one night and was pleased to hear the singing of a seductive water nymph. When he caught sight of her—green curls surrounded her beautiful face and she wore a blue garment—and reached for her to raise her veil, she pulled him into the depths. At the place where he disappeared, King Richard the Lionhearted found a flower, lovely as an undine—with fine green hair and a blue raiment of blossoms.

A further, very illustrative German name—"bride in hair" (in French *cheveux de Vénus* = "Venushair") is evidence that the change from being single to being married for women used to be associated with a change of hairstyle such as a different type of braiding or headgear. Up until the 18th century, it was a sign of virginity for distinguished brides to follow the custom of marrying "in hair," which means having undone, loosely hanging hair. This is described in the following German verse:

From the rather large, simple or filled, sometimes white but usually light-blue flowers that are similar in their shape to rose species like the "Persian Rose," "Miss Jekyll," or "Double Blue," the strongly puffed seed capsules develop. These can grow to be as large as a pigeon egg and have ovaries grown together to the tip with horizontally protruding pistils resembling horns. The German term of "capuchin herb" is probably based on this striking capuchin-like form and it could be further speculated whether the folksy English name of "devil-in-a-bush" can be explained by the fear of these many horns.

The seeds contained in the follicles are also black, triangular, and horizontally wrinkled. So their appearance could cause them to be easily mistaken for the seeds of the *Nigella sativa*. However, when they are ground the smell is less acrid than the *Nigella sativa*'s nutmeg or camphor smell. Instead, it tends to have the pleasant smell of strawberries or pineapples, which has also earned the plant the names strawberry cumin or pineapple cumin. The seeds tend to be used as a seasoning for sweet baked goods, as well as in the production of fruit ether and snuff.

The essential oil, represented with a proportion of 0.37% to 0.55%, possesses a pleasant smell and tastes like wild strawberries and is also vaguely reminiscent of musk-seed oil. The oil is yellow and fluoresces to a magnificent blue. This characteristic can also be used to help differentiate between the various black cumin seeds, which are often confused and mixed up with each other: in tests under filtered UV light, only the blue seed powder of *Nigella damascena* has a strong bluish fluorescence. In later chapters concerned with the cultivation areas and quality characteristics, there will be a more detailed look at the differences between the black cumin seeds.

A third botanic type should also be mentioned in greater detail here: **Nigella arvensis**, the field black cumin that is also called wild black cumin and oat or horse black cumin. This variety only reaches a height of up to 20 centimeters. The upright, hairless stem has branches starting at the bottom, taking the form of a small bush. It has alternating laciniated leaves and apical blossoms with a five-leaved flower cup that is light-blue with greenish stripes on the outside. The adnascene (growing together) of the 3 to 5 fruit leaves of the seed capsule only reaches up halfway. In contrast to the two other species, this is neither coarse nor puffed into a ball but tends to be longish with the little horns with which we are already familiar, earning it the scientific name of *Nigella arvensis cornuta*.

The seeds of the field black cumin are also black, somewhat coarse and triangular. When ground, they do not have the delicious smell of the more charming "love-in-a-mist" but tend instead to be reminiscent of the spicy, acrid character of the *Nigella sativa* seeds. Just like the latter, they are also used as a peppery spice and even for medicinal purposes. These are presumably the type of black cumin seeds that countryfolk use for fumigation against creeping vermin and poisonous animals—preferably against spiders, scorpions, and snakes. However, witches have also been mentioned within this context. Young German girls gave an unloved suitor the flowers as a gentle hint for him to "shove off"—this is why it bears the drastic German folk name of *schabab*, which means something like "scram" in English!

This now brings us to the borderline area where the field black cumin grows rampant in the grain fields as a "weed" and is fought accordingly. Although there is a reference in an older source that there is a species of black cumin that grows among the seeds in the coastal countries between the Mediterranean and the Black Sea, this apparently wasn't considered to be a plague. But since the German folk name

Radel (corn cockle) is equated with the Latin name *Nigella arvensis* in Zedler's *Encyclopedia*, this leads us to another clue: gracefully described as the corn carnation, carnation rose, or Our-Lady's Rose, the **corn cockle** is a genuine field weed in rye and wheat fields since the saponins it contains are actually poisonous and make the flour bitter. Even the name that St. Hildegard of Bingen used for the field black cumin, *Githerum ratde*, is an indication of such a confusion with the corn cockle, whose insidiously confusing botanic name is *Agrostémma **githago***. This name is composed of *agros*, "field," for the location; *stemma*, "garland," because of the round form of the flower; and *gith*, the old Arabian and Graeco-Roman name for *Nigella*. Other languages also demonstrate this shift of the name from black field cumin to corn cockle: the Italian name for the corn cockle is *gitto* and in French the *nigelle* becomes *nielle*—a true grain weed that causes *nielle du blé*, the "gout of the wheat."

The field black cumin has almost completely disappeared today, at least in Central Europe, as a result of extensive control measures.

The European Tradition—Part II

Equipped with these botanic tools, we can reassume the search for traces of the black cumin since the beginning of modern times and up into the present. At the same time, this is only meant to be a general survey of the history and propagation of this plant. Individual recipes from the German folk medicine will later be discussed in the chapter on special therapeutic applications, together with the experiences of the Arabian and Indian traditions, as well as more recent recommendations for use.

Hieronymus Bock's *New Kreutterbuch* (New Herbal Book) from the year 1539, as well as the quickly following compendia by his successors and imitators, are based on both the ancient sources, which we have already encountered, as well as the oral folk tradition that has become quite diversified in the meantime.

Nigella sativa, which has gradually multiplied itself into increasingly more species, can now be found once again as the "black domestic coriander," so that we can state the following: The Nigella species are now differentiated botanically between "domestic" (meaning cultivated) and "wild" varieties; in addition, one of these domestic sorts has apparently borrowed something from the coriander because of its apparent similarity with the narrow upper leaves of this spice plant. So the folk saying possibly had a justified influence on the classification of the taste.

Hieronymus Bock was the first to mention that the "most lovely Nigella," which is not hard to recognize as the *Nigella damascena*, "is planted in the pleasure gardens," where the smell and taste of the seeds began to weaken since they also increasingly grew wild. In contrast, *Nigella arvensis*, the actual wild black cumin or coriander, is botanically exposed as a "pseudo-melanthium." However, in terms of its medicinal effect, it is placed beside the "Melanthium sativum"—at least until the confusion with the corn cockle, as already mentioned, was to become its undoing...

About 200 years after Hieronymus Bock, the *New Complete Herbal Book* by Jacobus Theodorus Tabernaemontanus was published in 1731 as the last large German encyclopedia of medicinal plants. It offers the most comprehensive state of knowledge from this period, including information about the medicine herb and weed nigella. Although it bears the supplementary name of "coriander" or "melanthium" here, it is primarily called "nard herb" or "nard seed"—particularly fragrant plants have been called "nards" since time immemorial. There is also no longer mention of a *Nigella hispanica* or *Nigella cretica* as local plants since the advantages of the Bohemian *Nardus Bohemica* had been recognized by this time.

The various species were now differentiated only on the basis of botanic aspects and not according to their officinal effectiveness. All of the authors familiar with herbs recognized this curative power and also agreed that the seeds shouldn't be taken when they are green, in an excessive amount, or unnecessarily, since they otherwise could even have a harmful effect. There is also the occasional recommendation to not take the "fiery and dry" seeds in a dry state but only bake them in bread. When this is done, they develop an effect like that of coriander.

Melanthium Oleum, the oil pressed out of the black cumin seeds, is mentioned somewhat less frequently. The same applies to the *Oleum Nigellae*, the essential oil extracted in the classical manner through steam distillation. However, both of these oils should be given in a much more careful dosage than the seeds. The abundance of described applications and recipes basically corresponds to the knowledge about the "true nigella of the ancients" that has traditionally been handed down. At the beginning of his chapter about the "nard seeds," Tabernaemontanus writes:

> The ancients only described one genus; we are familiar with
> six different ones. Yet, they all have almost the same strength
> and effect, with one surpassing the others at most in terms of
> intensity and quality ...

However, he was definitely aware of the confusion between wild black cumin and the corn cockle since he even wrote the following about the seeds of the nigella:

> Many doctors and apothecaries use the seeds of the corn cockle
> in place of this nard seed, and although this error has been
> clarified by educated men and is now "as clear as the bright
> sun at noon," there are still so many people inexperienced in
> the knowledge of herbs who are so obstinate in this error that
> they cannot be talked out of it.

Did this fateful error contribute to such a popular medicinal and spice plant like the black cumin having been almost completely forgotten in Europe for centuries? Since, on the other hand, it never lost its legendary fame in the Orient, from

Egypt to Syria and Turkey to India and China, there may be a further possible explanation, which will be investigated in the following chapter.

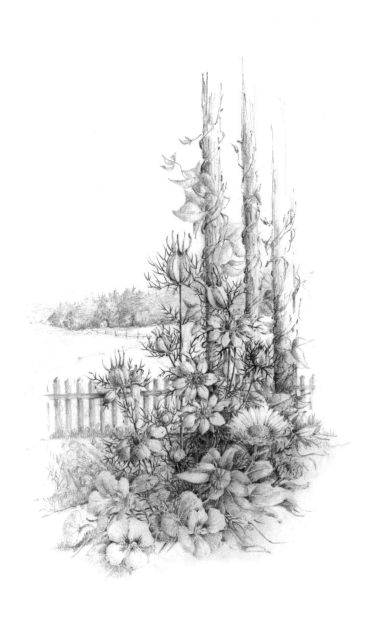

What Happens When Seeds Go on a Journey?

The Probable Consequences of a Transplantation
Considering the degree of familiarity that the black cumin enjoyed in earlier times even in the Central-European latitudes as a spice and medicinal plant, the question naturally arises whether the mysterious seeds were imported from the Orient. However, there is much to be said against this idea: their use by the simple folk as a bread seasoning and as an apparently constantly available home remedy; the self-sowing of the plant seeds that led to increasingly greater propagation as well as to the plant growing wild; and ultimately also the notorious confusion of the varieties with each other. If we investigate more closely, a number of scientific studies state that *Nigella damascena* was not only an ornamental garden plant and appeared in a wild form on compost heaps and at dumps, but that it was also cultivated and grown on the fields in Central Europe already at the beginning of the 16th century. The use of black cumin as a spice may have been the primary reason for this, yet the earlier official use as a remedy on the basis of the essential oil's effective ingredients has been proved in studies on medicinal-plant culture and the herb trade. A further factor here is the use of German-Damascene strawberry black cumin for the aromatization of sweets, delicious fruit tarts, liqueurs, and even snuff.

The field cultivation of both sorts in Germany has primarily been proved in the area around the city of Erfurt. In a book from the first half of the 20th century, the cultivation methods were described in detail. It states that the plant prefers light, loamy soils without fresh fertilization. It was sowed in spring as of March or as a subsequent crop in autumn. Around the end of August, the seeds were ripe, which could be recognized by the dark coloration of the seed capsules. After the harvest, the plants were bundled and left on the ground for a number of days so that the seeds could continue to ripen. When the stem and leaves were dried out, they were threshed like grain and stored in a cool and dry place.

This essentially corresponds to the current cultivation and processing methods for black cumin in North Africa, West Asia, and India. However, when we consider that this sun-pampered plant thrives best in areas that are very warm and have little rainfall, preferring a light, sandy soil, the question does arise whether the climatic and soil conditions in central Germany are or were suitable for an optimal development of the powerful components in the long run. Only dry, airy environmental influences can produce such pinnated, "airy" leaves, as the herbal pastor Weidinger has so aptly expressed it. However, the seeds are effected even more intensely by external conditions. Even in the old sources, the characterization of the plant ranges from "warm and dry in the second degree" to "fiery and dry in the third degree." When more than half a dozen species of black cumin that are most frequently used for medical purposes are listed in Zedler's *Encyclopedia* (18th century), this insightful advice is included as well:

The seeds are needed as medicine
And these are prescribed from Italy
Since they are much better than those
That usually grow in Germany

In the northern countries, the yield of seeds is distinctly lower and the plant grows considerably more poorly in salty or acidic soils. For this reason, it's no wonder that the Syrian black cumin seeds that were sowed in Germany as a test some years ago produced plants with less strength; the seeds were smaller and more wrinkled. Corresponding tests with Egyptian seeds established that they had a very poor rate of germination. At the same time, this tells us that a German *Nigella damascena* that has been transplanted from the Mediterranean or Mesopotamia to the German river meadows of Unstrut and Saale or in the country gardens of the

Rhineland must differ considerably from the original "true" Syrian plant in its effectiveness as well. As a comparison, we can imagine what effects transplanting a southern type of grape to the north would have on the wine!

How Tradition and Modern Times Work Together

Interesting Facts About Cultivation, Seed Extraction, and Oil-Pressing

Today black cumin is primarily cultivated in Egypt, the Sudan, and Ethiopia, some Mediterranean countries, Syria and Turkey, Irak, Iran, Pakistan, and India. Because of the great demand in the West, the USA has recently also became a cultivation nation. Ideal growth circumstances prevail in most of these countries, namely a warm, very sunny and dry climate, as well as suitable soil conditions, so that the plant can optimally develop the powerful components in its seed capsule. Heavy, rich soils or cold weather are not beneficial to the plant and the danger of fungus infection and other plant pests increases with too much humidity in the air. Up to now, cultivation has still taken place, as far as we know, largely under traditional conditions; this is often also called "*conventional* cultivation" in the product descriptions. At least the economic circumstances alone cause an adherence to organic or biological principles; there isn't (yet) "*controlled* organic cultivation" in these countries, even if some product descriptions would like to suggest this to the consumer.

With increasingly modern research and scientific study of black cumin, its application possibilities and effects, knowledge about appropriate methods of cultivation and the extraction of oil has become more diversified. Black cumin can do without chemicals from the time of sowing to final processing if certain rules are taken into consideration. In the extraction of the oil, cold-pressing and protection from oxidation is particularly important.

37

Black cumin is an annual plant. The time for sowing is dependent on the country and warm temperatures. This usually takes place between September and November, but can also extend into the winter. In Syria, for example, the sowing period lasts up into February. Depending on the region, there are also countries with two harvests, in the spring and in autumn. The plants are watered until blossoming time but then no longer after this time when the fruit capsules begin to form so that the seeds stay dry. In summer, mostly in July, the harvest can take place after the bloom as soon as the capsules turn dark and, although the plants are still green, the leaves are beginning to die from the bottom up—a certain sign that the power of the plant is now being given to the seed capsules.

The plants are cut with a sickle 5 centimeters above the ground. It is important that they are cut in the evening or before sunrise so that no dew is on them. References to certain phases of the moon for the harvest time are also found occasionally. The plants are then bundled and spread to dry on large cloths in the shade. During this time, the plant bundles should be turned over now and then. After about one week, the seed capsules spring open on their own and the seeds can be threshed, like grain. The procedure that follows depends upon whether the whole seeds are to be sold or whether oil is to be pressed on site or in the consumer country.

In Egypt, black cumin is grown on large field areas in the south around the Upper Nile, as well as in selected oases in the middle of the Arabian desert. The interest of the health-conscious West, where black cumin oil is primarily used as a food supplement and is tested by way of corresponding analyses, should offer good motivation for cultivation "according to organic principles." However, in Germany there are test results for a black cumin oil of Egyptian origin distributed through health-food stores and natural-foods stores that still show evidence of pesticidal residue, even if it is at a minimal level.

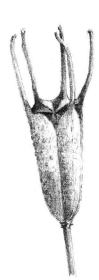

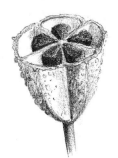

Cross-section of the
seed capsule
(collective follicular fruit)

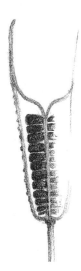

Seed capsule
(enlarged) of the
Nigella Sativa

Longitudinal section
of the seed capsule

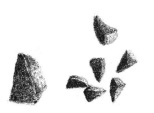

Black cumin seeds (triangular
and horizontally wrinkled)

An article about the "secret of the Pharaohs" may be even more thought-provoking as it enthusiastically reports about the ancient oil-presses with mashing stones made of rose granite and wooden hand presses. This awakens romantic images of an archaically simple and holistically rounded life, but says nothing about the hygienic circumstances under which the highly sensitive black cumin seeds are pressed to make the very susceptible oil. The same applies to the conditions for filtering and filling it into containers, for storage, and for transportation.

Cold-Pressing without Solvents

Even if the black cumin seeds already naturally contain all the valuable components that are concentrated in both its fatty oils and its essential oils, a person would have to eat quite a great many seeds in order to achieve an effect equivalent to that of taking one teaspoon of oil. In order to produce black cumin oil in the quality required of a food supplement, the native oil must be extracted through cold-pressing, although the yield is less than through other methods. Otherwise, valuable unsaturated fatty acids would be destroyed by the higher temperatures. It is also obvious that this must be a "first-pressing," whereby neither the "oil cake" of crushed grist residue is allowed to be washed out one more time nor the native cold-pressed oil "stretched" with oils of a less recommended quality.

In the customary oil-pressing, organic or chemical solvents are used for the extraction process. In a book about black cumin that was published in Egypt a number of years ago, oil-extraction methods such as those using a solvent like hexane, an ingredient of petroleum, were described: the crushed black cumin seeds are put into a large container filled with hexane (petroleum) for six to eight hours and kept in constant movement. Heating the mixture to 35° – 40° C (according to other sources, the temperature can even reach 60° C) causes the hexane (petroleum) to volatilize and the *fatty* oil remains. The *essential* oil is then extracted through a steam-distillation process. The thought of a food supplement created in such a way is ... hmm, what's your opinion about it?

In order to exclude such an element of uncertainty, some importers bring the seeds to the country where the oil is to be sold in order to have the pressing supervised. This guarantees that the oil is cold-pressed and doesn't suffer a loss of quality because of pouring it from container to container a number of times. However, the long transportation route and the storage problems still exist since not only the oil but also the black cumin seeds themselves are highly sensitive to environmental influences and susceptible to oxidation (just think of nuts that have become rancid!).

The Dangers of Oxygen

Oxidation occurs when atmospheric oxygen attacks double bonds in the unsaturated fatty acids, causing their structure to change. In this process, fatty acids with less digestible characteristics such as erucic acid or behenic acid can be created and the positive effect of a vegetable fat or oil with a high proportion of essential fatty acids may not only be reduced but even become harmful. In addition, the formation of peroxide causes the creation of unstable oxygen molecules, known as free radicals, that can have the effect of damaging tissue and are seen to be related to many health disorders.

The analysis of the peroxide value gives us information about the degree of oxidation. It shows how much milligram-equivalent oxygen is detectable in 1000 grams of a substance. It denotes the amount of peroxides created through oxidation and thereby the condition of freshness for an oil or fat, as well as being an indication of the loss of potency for the fat's own antioxidants.

Oxidation can be prevented or at least strongly reduced by the exclusion of oxygen or addition of antioxidants. Antioxidants are organic compounds, such as tocopherols like vitamin E, that can protect oils and fats from undesired changes.

In the case of black cumin, an oxidation of seeds and oil can be reduced by the following safety measures:

- Oil-pressing according to modern procedures with the exclusion of oxygen in order to reduce oxidation processes and thereby the decomposition of valuable substances as far as possible:
- Treatment of the oil with nitrogen and the addition of vitamin E (however, this must be minimal since the opposite effect will otherwise occur) as antioxidants:

- Use of transportation containers consisting of an especially suited material and filled with an inert gas (nitrogen, carbon dioxide);
- Filling the containers *completely* with the sensitive transport commodity;
- Making sure there is an exclusion of light;
- Providing cool and dry storage.

In the comparison between two "organic varieties" of Egyptian black cumin oil distributed in Germany, it was determined that the cold-pressed oil produced entirely in Egypt had a higher peroxide value (82.76) than the other type, for which the seeds had been transported to Germany and pressed into oil there (61.14). This difference could also be recognized in the purer taste and a higher degree of digestibility.

However, the advantages of pressing the oil in Germany are offset by disadvantage that the seeds cannot be pressed fresh from the harvest and it therefore isn't possible to filter and draw off the oil immediately. Experts consider the ideal situation to be when the cultivation area and the pressing procedure are located close to each other so that no unnecessary storage times and long transportation routes occur during this stage. This can guarantee better protection against oxidation, as well as higher quality. A black cumin oil that was also tested fulfills these preconditions and had the lowest peroxide value (34.86) in comparison to the other two. A peroxide value of this magnitude can be seen as typical for *Nigella sativa* and insures that no spoilage of fat has occurred. This oil tastes pleasantly mild, without the "aftertaste" that is often typical of the oil, is well-tolerable, and still very effective. However, it doesn't come from Egypt but Syria.

Personal Experience Counts

The Syrian Model Example

Syria is also a classic cultivation country for black cumin. The best quality crops thrive here in the north between the Euphrates and the Tigris (the old Assyrian "Mesopotamia") and in Houran, which is 80 to 90 kilometers south of Damascus. The entire region is free of environmental pollution through industry and, instead of being the exception, traditional "organic" cultivation is the rule. The soils here are completely free of toxins and do not suffer from the effects of a monoculture. It is important to also emphasize this fact since monoculture is connected with a one-sided exploitation of the nutrients in the soil and usually with the application of chemical fertilizers. These are absorbed by the plants and then reach the metabolism of human beings. Chemical additives in food can only be broken down very slowly by the body, if at all, and are deposited in the cellular tissue as waste products. The advantages of organic cultivation, which also includes crop rotation and letting the fields lay fallow, are therefore obvious.

In addition to the favorable starting conditions in our Syrian example, there is also the "holistic" concept. This means the supervision of all the steps, starting with the choice of seeds according to strict criteria and a natural manner of cultivation that is completely free of chemicals in selected locations, up to a careful cold-pressing and filling with the exclusion of oxidation, is in all in the same hands. This task has been undertaken by Dr. Diab Refai, M.D. with great expertise and a conscientious approach. In his homeland of Syria, he is personally familiar with the suppliers from whom he receives the seeds, as well as the farmers under contract and the cultivation areas. The seeds, which are stored only briefly after the harvest, are processed into the above-mentioned oil with a machine especially imported from Germany for the purpose of cold-pressing in a special procedure that excludes oxidation.

43

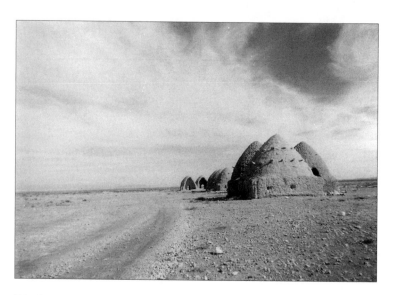

Black cumin cultivation area in Syria

The Turkish Model Example

True black cumin, *Nigella sativa*, has also been cultivated in Turkey for many centuries in that country's traditional manner. A series of black cumin species, which are indigenous to Asia Minor, grow wild in Turkey. The "true black cumin" is preferably cultivated in central Anatolia in the vicinity of the city of Konya, as well as along the Aegean Sea near Izmir. The conditions for growing black cumin are practically ideal in Turkey since it offers locations that are warm and not too wet and the soil is neither too light nor too heavy.

Dependent on the soil conditions and the climate from region to region, two harvests are common here: the first sowing in October can be harvested as of springtime and the second sowing in May is then harvested in August. In places where the blessings of progress (from the West) haven't yet arrived, cultivation takes place according to the simple agricultural survival patterns. Instead of monocultures and large field areas, this means in small fields with crop rota-

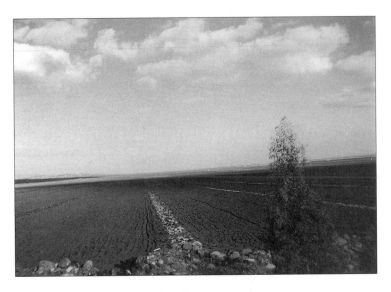

Syrian black cumin field shortly after sowing

tion, such as the succession of chickpeas, black cumin as an intercrop, and then lentils. Black cumin thrives best here in the second or third yield after chickpeas since nitrogen reaches the soil as a "fertilizer" in a natural way through the leguminous plants. The small farmers, who usually work as a family operation, use their own, botanically determined, non-treated seeds of the *Nigella sativa*. Cultivation experiments lasting several years in greatly differing regions have proved that Turkish seeds possess a high degree of germinability. On the basis of economic reasons alone, the use of artificial fertilizer or the purchase of herbicides or pesticides is not possible in the country's traditional manner of land utilization. We can therefore speak of *traditional cultivation* in a positive sense.

After the maturity of the seeds, they are usually still threshed by hand and the seeds are cleaned with simple fan installations. The oil is then pressed immediately. Screw presses operated by pressure are most frequently used, but hydraulic cylinder presses also may be employed. Solvents

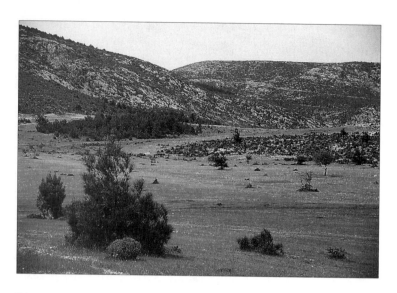

Black cumin cultivation area in Turkey

are not used, and the oil is just filtered mechanically. The black cumin oil extracted in this manner corresponds to the quality terms of "first-pressing" and "cold-pressed." Lesser qualities are extracted through the addition of cheaper "oil cake" (for example, palm-kernel fat or soybean grist) and used for industrial purposes. Cold-pressed black cumin oil develops just a low temperature in the screw press. The oil does not need to be stabilized or preserved with synthetic substances. It is naturally cloudy and therefore needs to be shaken before use.

On the basis of the growing demand from the West, the small Turkish farmers and oil producers themselves are interested in the proper time for the harvest and a clean extraction of oil. They are quite aware that the international trade has strict quality regulations and that, for example, first-class oil does not tolerate any air since it will otherwise oxidize. For this reason, the Turkish black cumin oil is immediately sealed into air-tight barrels after the pressing. A properly filled, "dry" oil, meaning without moisture, also doesn't contain any bacteria.

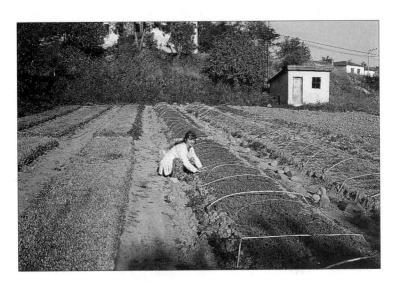

Renate Spannagel observes the cultivation of seedlings at the national testing farm in Turkey

Renate Spannagel, a German lecturer on herbs and expert on Turkey who, above all in Anatolia, has become very familiar with the land and mentality of the people through longer visits, has organized a project with the objective of supporting the small farmers there through "fair trade" and simultaneously having the certainty of a black cumin oil with first-class quality. She has achieved this by having the corresponding analyses done of both the fatty oil and the essential black cumin oil in Germany, which determine the fatty acid spectrum, the essential components, the microbiological purity, and the peroxide value, among other things. Particularly the peroxide value of 31 is an indication of very good quality and the necessary care in pressing, transporting, and storing the oil. A Turkish essential black cumin oil from the "entire plant" is also offered for sale.

In terms of her approach, Renate Spannagel says:

"Since the old tradition of black cumin cultivation has been promoted for centuries according to the traditional conditions of the country, it was a challenge for me to connect the Oriental culture with Western standards. At the same time, it is always a tightrope walk to show respect for the Oriental mentality and still achieve the Western demands for purity..."—an experiment that apparently has proved to be successful!

Most of the case histories included in the chapter on "Therapeutic Applications and Special Selected Recipes" are based on experiences with the above-mentioned black cumin oil of Syrian origin, but they naturally are not limited to it. There are also very positive, personally authentic experiences with the Turkish black cumin oil that have flowed into some of the special recipes. This correction also needs to be stated since some new publications propagate the misleading opinion that *Nigella sativa* is equivalent to **Egyptian** black cumin alone—a viewpoint unknown to the Oriental perspective—and that only this species is significant as a medicinal plant or that particularly rich and valuable components of the black cumin are chiefly developed in the Egyptian areas of cultivation. To date there have been no differences that are well-founded and demonstrable through analysis discovered between the Egyptian, Syrian, and Turkish black cumin oil in relation to such factors as the fatty acid spectrum, for example. The sole recognizable differences, such as the peroxide value, are associated with the care and attention given by the people to the use of a very sensitive plant. How else should it be possible that a plant of more than 3000 years in God's great garden could restrict its growth to a clear-cut district within certain national boundaries?

BLACK CUMIN: HOW IT WORKS—WHY IT HEALS

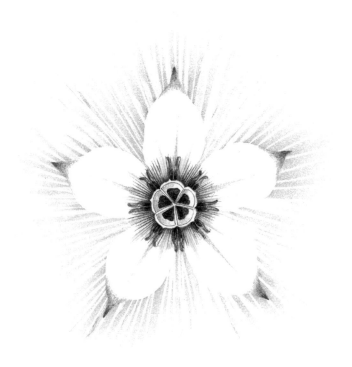

The Most Effective Components

Of the more than one-hundred components in the seeds of the black cumin, which has the effect of a complex remedy, many have not yet been researched or exhaustively researched today. However, some of the therapy successes cannot completely be explained on the basis of the substances known up to now. Instead, it may be possible to trace the effect to a "synergy effect" of the ingredients in the fatty oil and in the essential oil, as well as some trace elements. About 6% of the components are still largely unknown, and it may be that one or more highly effective factors are concealed here.

Black cumin seeds contain approximately 20% protein, 35% carbohydrates, and 35% to 45% vegetable oils and fats; the share of the essential oil consists of between 0.5% and 1.5%. The fatty acids proved to be in the fatty oil of the black cumin are up to 50% polyunsaturated and therefore "essential" for human beings. In addition, two particularly important individual active ingredients are the saponin *melathin* and the bitter principle *nigellin*; both of these are mutually responsible for the digestant and generally eliminating effect, which can also be used for gentle intestinal cleansing. It has also been possible to prove the existence of tannins in the seeds.

Moreover, a Turkish study by the University of Ankara mentions that the component *beta-sitosterol* has been isolated in a phytochemical analysis; along with linoleic acid, it is even called the most important active ingredient in black cumin oil. Sterols are aromatic alcohols that can be of either animal or vegetable origin. Interestingly enough, among other things beta-sitosterol, as a plant sterol, is known for sinking the cholesterol level (cholesterol, the best-known sterol there is), is of animal origin. In addition, beta-sitosterol is generally secretagogue (supports secretion).

Among other things, the anti-inflammatory, bronchodilating, and generally pain-relieving effect is attributed to some of the essential active ingredients, which are primarily *nigellone* and *thymoquinone* here; however, they must share this advantage with the polyunsaturated fatty acids, which play a truly *essential* role in the regulation of the overall metabolism and production of hormones.

The Fatty Oil

The fatty oil pressed out of the black cumin seeds with an excellent quality contains more than 80% unsaturated fatty acids. Oleic acid, a single unsaturated fatty acid with a share of 20 to 25%, and linoleic acid, a polyunsaturated fatty acid with a share between 50% and 60%, can be mentioned in this regard. During recent years, evening primrose oil and borage oil have become known because of their high content of polyunsaturated fatty acids and their resulting curative effect. Black cumin oil can be compared with them, yet it has further components and their uniquely favorable composition has a different synergetic and even more versatile effectiveness.

The fats contained in foods are compounds of various fatty acids with glycerin. According to their molecular structure, saturated fatty acids are divided into simple bonds that tend to be "slow to react" and single or polyunsaturated fatty acids that can enter into new compounds with other substances through double bonds and play an important role for numerous vital functions. Put into pictorial terms, the saturated fatty acids are those "marriageable," single unsaturated fatty acids are the "monogamously married," and polyunsaturated fatty acids are "polygamous" or married to two, three, or four partners. When two unsaturated double bonds are located next to each other, as is the case for the linoleic acid, for example, these powers add up into a so-called "electron cloud"; this should be understood as a special electrical charge that produces a new charging of the living substance within the organism.

Those polyunsaturated fatty acids that are vital and must be supplied to the body, primarily from fats and oils of plant origin, are also called essential fatty acids. In strict terms, only the linoleic and the linolenic acids are included here since these cannot be created by the organism while the highly unsaturated arachidonic acid can also be synthetically formed from linoleic acid within the body. In black cumin oil, the high portion of up to 60% linoleic acid, which has been proved by analyses, provides for this. In addition, important hormone-like substances are created as an intermediate stage through the gamma-linoleic acid on the way to this biosynthesis of the body—the *prostaglandins*, which play a special role in the regulation of the immune system. There will be more about this later since we first want to deal with the diverse tasks of the unsaturated fatty acids in the body, as well as the consequences caused by a deficiency of them.

The Essential Fatty Acids

The unsaturated fatty acids are among the vital building blocks of the cells, particularly the cell membranes and vesicular breathing. They are indispensable for the membrane function, for the development and function of the brain and central nervous system, as well as for undisturbed growth. They play a significant role in the transportation of oxygen into the cells and for its storage in the cell membrane. As an important factor for the inner breathing, they also have an effect against oxidation, as well as a lack of oxygen and reduced vesicular breathing. This is considered to be a favorable medium for the anomalous development of bacteria into pathogenic germs: when harm takes place over a longer period of time, the cell becomes a fermenting cell and the respiratory exchange becomes a fermentation exchange—this is also seen to be a factor in the occurrence of cancer.

In contrast to the saturated fatty acids with their straight form and sticky consistency, and the trans-fatty acids that occur through processes of heating and hardening, the crooked form of the unsaturated fatty acids has the effect that they cannot cluster with each other, are slippery, and the arteries do not become clogged. They have the quality of spreading out in very thin layers, which is called surface activity. This is, for example, the basis for the possibility of transporting toxins to the surface of the skin, where it can be eliminated and removed.

The unsaturated fatty acids also play an important role in the maintenance and activation of a regulated metabolism. For example, they make sure that there is an adequate burning of the fat and protein in the body cells. This applies primarily to the transformation of the saturated fatty acids, which mainly come from animal fats, whereby they work against the depositing of surplus fats in tissue. Moreover, disorders in the fat metabolism based on an insulin deficiency can be balanced and an elevated cholesterol level in the blood can be lowered. Through the increase of the bile secretion, gallbladder disorders and a functional weakness of the liver can be favorably influenced. Positive effects on the blood circulation, as well as the hormone and immune system, have also been determined.

A deficiency of such essential building substances must inevitably lead to health disorders. It was proved that infants who received synthetically produced baby food with a lower content of essential fatty acids instead of mother's milk during a study carried out in the 1950s were found to have dry, scaly skin with a tendency towards eczemas and rashes—symptoms that soon disappeared with the addition of essential fatty acids. Through further studies, including those with adults, it was possible to prove that such a deficiency not only leads to the formation of skin scales, psoriasis, and abscesses, but also can cause growth inhibitions and disorders of the central nervous system.

On the basis of their molecular structure, essential fatty acids more easily enter into compounds with other substances. Within the body they are converted into extremely active substances in the metabolic processes. This brings us to the fascinating topic of *prostaglandins*, hormone-like substances that are considerably involved in contributing to the rediscovered renown of black cumin oil through their regulation of the immune system and hormone system, which means in the treatment of allergic symptoms and the premenstrual system, for example.

The Prostaglandins

The Nobel Prize for Medicine was awarded in 1982 for research on the prostaglandins. At the same time, people spoke of the possibility of bringing about a revolution through the prostaglandins in both biology and the field of practical medicine. Has this proved to be true?

The *prostaglandins* are not just evident in the prostata, as the name would suggest, but within the entire organism. However, they are contained in the greatest concentration in sperm and mother's milk. They are not stored in the organism but released through nerve stimulation or messenger substances, have just a short lifespan, and have the effect of "tissue hormones" on the cells in their immediate vicinity. The organism forms them on the spot and only when they are necessary. Since essential fatty acids participate in their creation to a large degree, an increased supply of suitable vegetable oils and fats can effectively support this synthesis undertaken by the body.

More than one-dozen prostaglandins, which generally play an important role for the function of the blood and the entire metabolism, have already become known up to this day. However, their effect is not just positive, as is often and readily imparted, but can also be just the opposite since there are two different types of prostaglandins: the first series have an anti-inflammatory effect and protect the cells, while the second series even promotes and maintains inflammatory processes. It is undisputed that prostaglandin E1 is a highly active substance with a favorable influence on the regulation of numerous bodily functions in connection with the immune system, hormone system, and nervous system. Among other things, this occurs through the effect on the excretion of hormones, messenger substances, and mucoids, the normalization of the vesicular respiration, and the control of the smooth musculature (bronchial tubes, blood pressure, uterus, etc.).

In order to describe it in simpler terms, prostaglandin E1 is created within the body through the biochemical conversion of cis-linoleic acid to gamma-linolenic acid and dihomo-gamma-linolenic acid as intermediate steps. The valuable gamma-linolenic acid, although present in mother's milk, is otherwise very rarely observed in nature. For example, it can be found in the plant seeds of the evening primrose and the stems and leaves of the borage. Since the linoleic acid taken in with the food, just like some vitamins, possesses no biological activity of its own, certain enzymes are required for the conversion into gamma-linolenic acid as a metabolically active substance. When there is an inhibition in the formation of enzymes, which is often caused by such disruptive factors as an improper diet, allergens, as well as psychological strain and the aging process, the corresponding counter-measures must be provided at any cost. An adequate supply of vitamin B, vitamin C, and the trace elements manganese, copper, and especially zinc is important so that the body can produce, above all, prostaglandins of the first series like prostaglandin E1 from the gamma-linolenic acid.

How Prostaglandin E1 Works

Prostaglandin E1

- Has a regulating effect on the brain functions, nerve conduction, and release of transmitter substances and messenger substances
- Contributes to lowering the blood pressure and vasodilation and prevents the clumping of the little blood platelets (thrombocytes)
- Regulates the immune system and activates the T- lymphocytes, which are essential for the body's defense against illness
- Inhibits allergic processes

- Normalizes inflammed skin
- Has a bronchodilating effect
- Increases hormonal secretion for the thyroid hormone and insulin, for example
- Regulates the female sexual hormones, above all during the corpous-luteum phase of the cycle, pregnancy, and menopause
- Has an anti-inflammatory effect by preventing the release of certain enzymes, as well as prostaglandins of the second series, which participate or are said to participate in the creation of inflammations.

Prostaglandins Are Not Always the Same

Prostaglandins are substances that have been discovered relatively recently, and their mode of action has not yet been completely researched. Even the specialized literature contains contradictions about the effect of prostaglandin E2 and arachidonic acid, which participates in its formation. However, a pharmacological study undertaken in 1994 by the King's College in London has come up with evidence that black cumin oil has a selectively inhibitory effect on some enzymes and therefore on the synthesis of certain prostaglandins. As a result, it can counter-act inflammatory processes like rheumatism, arthritis, and bronchial asthma.

When the linoleic acid within the body is converted through biosynthesis by way of gamma-linolenic acid into di-homo-gamma linolenic acid, either prostaglandin E1 is synthesized directly or prostaglandin E2 is synthesized through an additional intermediate step, arachidonic acid. Even if arachidonic acid, which occurs in peanut oil and fats of an animal origin, is taken in by the body directly with the food, prostaglandins of the second series are formed from it. These play a role in inflammatory processes, the occurrence of fever, and pain processes. The related leucotrines, which are created from the arachidonic acid as well, are also involved in the occurrence of such diseases as bronchial asthma. More recent research has even related them to the activation of the "free radicals" and therefore with possible cell damage. "Heavy stuff" like cortisone preparations are used to inhibit the release of the arachidonic acid. It's therefore no wonder that specialized literature contains the information that an increase of prostaglandin production is not particularly "desirable" ...

Since scientific studies have proved the pain-killing and anti-inflammatory effect of black cumin oil, and it is also recommended specifically for the treatment of rheumatic pain and stiffness in the joints, of bronchial asthma and eczema, in our search for traces we once again face a familiar puzzle here—all the more since each of the fatty acids mentioned is included among the omega-6 fatty acids because of the similar structure of their molecule chains.

However, there appear to be at least two ways out of this dilemma, as shown by further studies:

- Cell hormones, also including prostaglandins, that are formed primarily from the arachidonic acids occurring in animal fats have the effect of promoting various disease processes. On the other hand, if they have been produced through the biochemical conversion from fatty acids originating in vegetable oils and fats, they then inhibit such inflammatory processes. Tests have even demonstrated that the arachidonic metabolism can be inhibited through the special composition of other unsaturated fatty acids found in black cumin oil and possibly through their interaction as well. Through an adequate supply of linoleic and gamma-linolenic acid, as well as the supportive effect of vitamin B, vitamin C, and zinc, the very desirable formation of prostaglandin E1 can be influenced.
- Black cumin oil wouldn't be a complex remedy that deserves this name if it didn't have its own natural controls made from its components and built in to guard against the creation of undesirable side effects. Among these is *thymoquinone,* a main constituent of the essential oil that also has the effect of an antioxidant. Tests of the Pharmacology Group at King's College in London (1994), in

which thymoquinone was isolated from black cumin oil, were able to prove a selective inhibition of exactly those enzymes that are substantially involved within the body in the biosynthesis of certain "undesired" prostaglandins.

Of course, black cumin oil develops an effect here that is about five to ten times weaker than the concentrated component thymoquinone; yet, since its proportion is only 0.15 to 0.20%, either other substances in the oil must have the same effect and/or thymoquinone interacts synergetically with other components. This applies to both the inhibition of prostaglandin formation and the antioxidative efficacy.

Now that we have become familiar with thymoquinone as one constituent of the essential oil, we should take a closer look at the latter.

The Essential Oil

The essential oil is made by applying steam distillation to the seed. Between two and three-and-a-half kilograms of essential oil can be distilled from one ton of black cumin seed. We have only recently become aware of it in Central Europe along with the popularity of black cumin itself, although it has already been known in the ancient Indian teaching of Ayurveda, as well as in the classic French aromatherapy, where it has been classified with the anti-inflammatory and allergy-relieving (antihistamine) oils. The essential black cumin oil can be used in a great variety of ways, not only for fragrance lamps but also for massages, compresses, rub-downs, baths, and inhalations. Its effect extends beyond the purely physical level. If at all possible, be sure not to purchase a so-called "fractional" oil (in such a case it has only had the significant components drawn out of it) but an essential oil made from the "entire plant." This means that it has been made from all the volatile components of the respective plant parts, as is the case with the Turkish-quality essential black cumin oil, for example.

Black cumin contains 0.5% to 1.5% essential oil, giving the oil its unmistakably spicy smell and taste. Just like the fatty oil, the essential oil of black cumin has a golden yellow color but is lighter and naturally has a much more intensive smell. Among the components are sesquiterpenes (alpha-pinene and beta-pinene), savines and savinhydrates, phenoles (thymol and carvacrol), ketones (carvon), oxides (1.8-cineoles), terpene-alcohols (terpineol, borneol, linalool), and further constituents, of which two are particularly important: *thymoquinone*, which has already been mentioned, and *nigellone semohiprepinon.*

As is no surprise for nigella, various lists of essential components result in considerable differences. For example, an Indian study mentions a carvon content of 45 to 60%, but other sources only quote it to be 4%. The same applies to p-cymonen, which is stated to be 77% here but isn't mentioned by other sources. These contradictions can hardly be completely resolved without a doubt by attributing them to the different plant species or variations in the biochemical terminology. The most recent analyses have crystallized so-called "peaks" from the important components, which are still unknown and could not be identified. In the same manner, according to the newest scientific findings nigellone is a mixture between di-thymoquinone and thymoquinone; this means that calling a component "nigellone" is basically imprecise since it consists of chemical compounds with which we are already familiar. However, because of a lack of other solutions, we will continue to use the term that has already been introduced here, "nigellone."

Nigellone then has a bronchodilating, anti-spasmodic, and warming effect—which are all qualities that are particularly recommended for treatment of disorders of the respiratory system, such as bronchial asthma and whooping-cough. In addition, it inhibits the secretion of histamines and could be a true alternative to remedies containing cortisone for some allergy sufferers, as proved in accordance with an Indian study from the year 1993.

Thymoquinone has an anti-inflammatory and pain-killing effect in general. In addition, its choleretic effect (meaning stimulation of bile production) has been proved, which emphasizes its significance for the fat metabolism and detoxification. Moreover, thymoquinone has antioxidant qualities.

A Turkish study by the Pharmacological Faculty at the University of Ankara from the year 1985 describes the effect of thymoquinone as bronchodilating, protective against asthma attacks, and as an anti-histamine in such a manner that it actually appears to be identical with the nigellone mentioned above. A further Turkish study, implemented at the Agricultural Faculty of the University of Erzurum in 1989, has also proved the anti-bacterial and—even if more weakly effective—anti-mycotic qualities of the essential black cumin oil. Above all, this is attributed to its component of thymoquinone. In the Near East, black cumin has traditionally been used for preserving food, such as in the preservation or marination of vegetables.

A Natural Antioxidant

Unstable oxygen molecules—free radicals—threaten not only the structure of unsaturated fatty acids in salad oil but can also do their destructive work within the body. They primarily originate when oxygen isn't burned completely. Each of us has them within our body cells. However, when they gain prevalence they react aggressively, attacking the cell membranes of organs, as well as the immune cells, and leading to oxidation processes in the cells, whose fatty substances then become "rancid." Illnesses like coronary heart disease and cataract, the occurrence of cancer, and a premature aging process are associated with them.

Free radicals form through metabolic processes and are activated by environmental poisons, injurious products (alcohol, tobacco, etc.), pesticides and other food additives, air pollution and UV radiation, medications, and many other factors. An effective defense against the attack of the free radicals are antioxidants, which are also called "radical catchers" because they "catch" them, chemically binding them within the body. Endogenous (the body's own) anti-oxidants (such as certain enzymes) can join forces with other substances coming from the outside that are supplied with the food to form an effective radical-catcher troop. Not only are vitamin E, vitamin C, and beta-carotene known to produce this effect, but also trace elements like selenium and bioflavonoids. How meaningfully a complex remedy like black cumin oil is structured and how good the components supplement each other and work together is shown, among other things, by its constituent thymoquinone, whose function as an "emergency brake" has already been described in the synthesis of prostaglandin.

Mental-Emotional Ray of Hope

Black cumin primarily serves as a remedy on the physical level, yet its regulating influence on the immune system, on the metabolism, and last but not least on the hormonal balance also has an impact in the mental and emotional realm. Above all, this also can be ascribed to the essential oil, which only contains the water-soluble substances of the plant's aromatic substance. The well-known holistic effect of essential oils on the body, mind, and soul occurs because the sense of smell triggers the release of hormones and messenger substances. Through the limbic system in the brain and the autonomous nervous system, these achieve a harmonization that not only has physical effects but mental, emotional, and psychological ones as well.

In India, black cumin is known for its stimulating, mood-lifting, and tonicizing effect on such problems as concentration difficulties, mental exhaustion, and age-related mental degeneration. Yet, at the same time it also has a balancing and stabilizing effect for sleep disturbances and hyperactivity in children. If the essential oil is burned in a fragrance lamp, it can brighten up the mood when there is a tendency towards depression. The herbal pastor Weidinger, who was particularly involved with "herbs for the soul," gave black cumin the nickname of "ray of hope" as its mental and emotional motto.

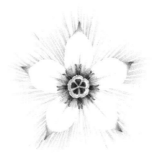

A Strong Combination:
Bitter Principles and Saponins

All nigella species contain the bitter principle *nigellin*. Oddly enough, research hasn't yet achieved clarity about whether or not this is an alkaloid, as it was previously assumed; on the other hand, for *damascenin*, a comparable active agent of Damascene cumin, this relationship appears to be proved.

The alkaloids are among the strongest active agents in plants, therefore often making them the most toxic and demanding of careful treatment. Among others, these occur in the nightshade, poppy plants, and crowfoot plants. In earlier times, they were common ingredients in the witches' kitchen since many of them can produce a consciousness-changing or narcotizing effect. One example of this is the alkaloid morphine that is found in the opium poppy. However, this is primarily meant to be a reminder that great care should already be taken in the selection of black cumin seeds, which naturally also applies to the dosage of every powerful curative remedy.

Because of its bitter principle nigellin, nigella has an activating effect on the appetite and digestion. It stimulates the digestive juices and enzymes in the stomach and intestines, also promoting the function of the liver and gallbladder. Alkaloids have also traditionally been known for their sudonific effect, as well as the stimulation of salivation. The medical world prefers to use them again chronic inflammation with the formation of stones on the basis of their anti-spasmodic effect. For example, the musculature of the bile ducts is relaxed in cases of gallstones, which supports increased bile secretion. Through the draining effect and promotion of kidney activity, excess acids within the body are also broken down. This leads to a great relief for the organism that helps reinstate the acid-alkaline balance and thereby eliminates the preconditions for a chronic susceptibility to infections. In addition, bitter principles are also said to influence the nervous system since they have a regenerating effect in cases of nervous exhaustion.

One further effective agent of black cumin, belonging to the large group of the glycosides, is the saponin *melanthin* (melanthingenin = hederagenin). As evident from the name, this is also an important component of the medicinal plant "Melanthium sativum" with a proportion of 1.5%. Saponins were given their name because they foam strongly in water and thereby have a certain similarity with soap. However, they don't have the latter's alkaline reaction. Because of their strong cleansing properties, they were already used in ancient times as a detergent and emulsifier because of their good solubility. With regard to inner cleansing, the folk medicine has proved their use as a laxative and emetic. Among other things, they are also medicinally significant because they have the effect of increasing solubility for the digitalis plants, which serve as cardiac stimulants. As a natural constituent in food, they promote the absorption of nutrients through the stimulation of the gastric juices.

Saponins have a strong local stimulating effect and serve to increase the amount of secretion. They are considered to be particularly mucolytic and expectorant, providing for a liquefaction of the bronchial secretion, as well as a quick removal of the bronchial mucus. Because of the increased secretion of gastric juices, they have a digestant, as well as diuretic effect. The frequently mentioned "blood-cleansing" effect may be related to this context, whereby in addition to a promotion of gland secretion and kidney elimination there is also an alternation of the organism's reactions to stimuli in cases of allergens, for example, which means the inclusion of the immune system. The old experiential art of healing has handed down the successful inner application of plants containing saponins for certain chronic skin diseases, particular eczema. However, this is still waiting for clinical study and official recognition. Because of the similarity of its structure with certain hormones within the body, it also has a regulating effect on the hormonal activities.

The saponin melanthin, as an important component of black cumin, supports bitter principle nigellin's diversely curative effects on the metabolism. This means that its effect is appetite-stimulating and digestant, generally cleansing, and eliminatory. The described effects on the respiratory system, as well as the immune system and hormone system, possess a great similarity to those of the prostaglandins, once again confirming the remarkable "synergy effect" of black cumin.

THE AREAS OF APPLICATION

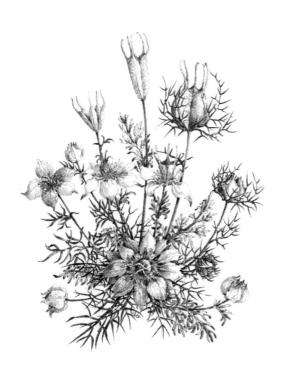

Traditional Experience and the Latest Research

Now that various of its most important components have been listed here, it should once again be emphasized that black cumin must be seen as a *complex remedy* in a twofold sense:

- The more than one-hundred components, some of which have not yet been adequately researched or are still unknown, complement each other to create a synergy effect. This means that their interaction not only adds up to the effect of the individual substances but also intensifies them through potentialization.
- In accordance with this, black cumin is not a "medicament" that has an isolated effect but develops an extremely broad range of action as a food supplement remedy.

The following qualities and curative effects of the black cumin have been handed down by the folk medicine of both the Near East and Europe:

- Digestant, carminative
- Slightly stimulating in general, stimulating for kidneys, diureticum, and calculi-dissolving (litholytic)
- Menstruation-promoting (emmenagogic), dilating, milk-promoting (lactiferous)
- Anti-inflammatory (also externally for wound-healing)
- Bronchodilatory, mucolytic (expectorant), anti-spasmodic, as well as relaxing for the nerves
- Anti-bacterial, anti-mycotic in a restricted manner
- Vermicidal
- Cleanses and smooths (externally for skin care)

The traditional use in cosmetics and hygiene (for example, as an insect repellent), as well as its use as a popular bread seasoning and kitchen spice should be particularly emphasized.

The traditions that have been handed down and modern research have unanimously substantiated the beneficial effect of black cumin for the following complaints and symptoms of disease, which can be treated in a supportive manner, as well as *a preventive measure.*

- Digestive complaints and related metabolic disorders: diseases of the gastrointestinal tract, gastritis, flatulence, diarrhea, inflammations of the liver, gallstones, kidney stones; raised cholesterol level; adult-onset diabetes (type II diabetes); also as a preventive measure for intestinal cleansing (for intestinal fungi like *Candida albicans*)
- Disorders of the immune system, which are mainly manifested in two forms:
  - Excessive allergic reactions like bronchial asthma, constant runny nose, hay fever, allergic conjunctivitis, neurodermitis, other skin diseases, and further related problems
  - Lowered immune resistance or immune weakness with symptoms like chronic susceptibility to infection, frequent colds, and other related problems
  - Respiratory disorders: bronchitis, stubborn hacking cough, whooping-cough, sinusitis, catarrhalic condition, lung diseases
- Disorders of the hormonal system
  - In women: menstruation disorders, particularly the premenstrual syndrome, menopausal complaints, headaches based on hormonal problems, and depression
  - In men: disturbance of potency
- Circulatory disorders and vascular diseases like hemorrhoids and varicose ulcers
- General decrease in vitality, concentration difficulties, sleep disturbances. Hyperactivity in children, forgetfulness caused by age

The following areas of application can additionally be mentioned for the primarily *external use* of black cumin oil:

- Skin diseases like acne, psoriasis, skin fungus, nettle rash, itching: also for impetigo, fistula, ulcers, tumors, and callosities; warts and thorn warts
- Loss of hair
- Contusions, bruises, effusions of blood, and wounds of all types
- Arthritis and rheumatic complaints
- Hemorrhoids.

In addition, modern science and research are currently working on studies investigating a possible inhibition of tumor growth through black cumin and thereby recommending its use within the scope of a supportive or preventive therapy for cancer. Similar research is also taking place for auto-immune diseases considered to be resistant to therapy, such as multiple sclerosis. Some newer therapy approaches will be covered later, but this is neither meant to propagate a new anticancer drug nor self-medication. This type of complex pathological process within the body can be explained on the basis of many and various causes, whereby we can be quite certain that a defective immune system always plays a role. As is particularly emphasized in almost all of the more recent studies, the regulating influence of black cumin on the immune system is the focus of its effectiveness; when this has been strengthened and stabilized, a variety of different health disorders can be simultaneously eliminated or at least relieved. In order to provide a better understanding of how and where a treatment with black cumin starts here, a brief description of the immune system's work for the body's defense appears necessary.

For Example: The Immune System

This Is How It Normally Functions ...

We can imagine our immune system to virtually have the form of a little state, for the preservation of which the blood circulation and the lymph system have set up mutual defensive troops with precisely determined scopes of duty. The red blood corpuscles (erythrocytes) have the peaceful function of transporting oxygen, while the white blood corpuscles (leucocytes) must be sure that they recognize, defend against, and, if necessary, also destroy attacking enemies. In a healthy human being, only about 10% of these defensive cells are active. They come out of their various resting places in the organs and glands only when the organism requires their help; in these types of emergency cases, they are even capable of reproducing themselves in their numbers.

Important defensive cells are the lymphocytes, which belong to the white blood corpuscles. Of these, the B-lymphocytes primarily produce antibodies while the T-lymphocytes with the subgroups of helper cells, killer cells, and phagocytes take over very specific functions in the body's own defense and are additionally controlled by suppressor cells. As we can see, this interaction is quite complicated and can easily become unbalanced when the division of labor not longer works: the immune system then gets on the wrong track and starts to act "crazy." This can be fundamentally expressed in two different types of disorders: lowered resistance of the immune system or a defensive reaction that is too intensive.

Weakened Immune Resistance

When too few antibodies are formed and the defensive cells are inferior in strength or number to the attacking microorganisms, we speak of lowered resistance. This can be initially expressed in a physical and vegetative exhaustion, then lead to a greater susceptibility to infection, and ultimately develop into chronic complaints. Viral infections on an increasingly frequent basis, the entire spectrum of respiratory disorders, as well as inexplicable pain in the stomach or skin rashes (because of fungal infection, for example) are danger signals for this type of weakened immune system.

When the immune system dysfunctions even further, the number of controlling suppressor cells multiplies excessively in relation to the active defensive cells and the body's defenses are increasingly switched off. This ultimately becomes an actual "immune blockage." The breeding ground for both chronic and malignant diseases has thus been created since malignantly changed cells can now spread unhindered when the body's defensive system is intensively weakened or has broken down.

Aggressive Immune Resistance

In the reverse case, the immune system's reaction can become too intensive and excessive, such as the situation expressed in allergic symptoms. When there is an intact immune system with the proper division of labor, the T-lymphocytes can distinguish between harmless and harmful substances. However, when there are too many helper cells but too few suppressor cells to control them, this is no longer the case. As a result, too much pathological immunoglobulin (IgE) is produced as an antibody, which connects with antigens (such as certain allergy-triggering protein substances in pollen) to form circulating immune complexes. However, when these occur in concentrations that are too high, they can no longer be eliminated by the phagocytes, which is normally the case, but turn against the body in a self-destructive manner. Immune complexes can also cause immune blockages, whereby an uncontrolled tumor growth is made possible in turn. Seen from this perspective, allergic disorders are auto-aggressive reactions.

... And This Is How Black Cumin Intervenes in a Regulatory Manner

Through an excessive immune reaction, inflammatory and rheumatic processes are triggered, among other things. But, above all, allergic symptoms are triggered that can be expressed in the form of asthma, hay fever, skin diseases, and the intolerance of certain foods. Because of many environmental factors that strain the immune system, today every fifth person—even every third or second according to some statistical information—suffers from an allergic disease.

To avoid the extremely disruptive and also frequently disfiguring symptoms, which also have a stronger relapse tendency, being treated solely on the surface and with a short-term effect, a therapy approach should get to the root of the matter and aim for a fundamental reorientation and regulation of the immune system as its most important task. This includes:

- The stabilization of the exaggerated defensive function of the T-lymphocytes or B-lymphocytes
- The increase of the suppressor cells to control the excessive IgE production
- The inhibition of allergy-triggering messenger substances in the body (so-called "allergy mediators"), like histamine
- With the participation of IgE, the elimination of immune complexes that are pathologically producing and occur in concentrations that are too high.

Is this possible at all? Because of both the beneficial synergetic interaction of its components and particularly because of the development of prostaglandin E1 from the essential fatty acids converted within the body, black cumin actually has a *possible* answer to offer as a response to many of these questions. To a high degree, prostaglandin E1 is an immune-regulatory substance, which is demonstrated in the anti-spasmodic and secretion-stimulating effect in cases of bronchial asthma, stubborn hacking cough, and constant runny nose. In addition, it triggers anti-inflammatory and vasodilatory reactions.

Recent research studies have confirmed the supposition that people suffering from allergies apparently require a greater supply of essential fatty acids, which is quite difficult through the normal consumption of foods. This is presumably also related to the situation of a defect in the fatty-acid metabolism, which can be explained by the deficiency or inadequate activity and therefore blockage of a specific enzyme, the delta-6-desaturase. The result of this within the body is an inadequate conversion of linoleic acid into gamma-linolenic acid and dihomo-gamma-linolenic acid, the necessary precursors for the development of prostaglandin E1. Many disruptive factors have been made responsible for this problem such as the aging process, psychological strains, allergens, as well as the consequences of improper diet, alcohol, and nicotine. Chronic seats of disease and viral infections can also contribute to this seemingly small, but grave dysfunction.

In black cumin's effect on the immune system, the participation of the essential substances, primarily nigellone and thymoquinone, should also be taken into consideration. They play an important role in respiratory diseases, especially in allergic forms like bronchial asthma and hay fever, and particularly support the anti-inflammatory, bronchodilatory, and secretagogic effect of prostaglandin E1.

In a similar manner, black cumin regulates the other main disorder in the body's own defense, *the weakened immune response*. An improper lifestyle and the additional strain caused by environmental conditions, which can also be called the "overall toxic situation," are substantially involved as the causes. The consequences of this can range from simple exhaustion and general weakness to chronic and more frequently occurring infectious diseases, skin rashes, mycosis, and inexplicable inflammations, up to cancer and AIDS (the virus-caused Acquired Immune Deficiency Syndrome) with a complete collapse of the immune system.

74

Every treatment of immune weakness has the goal of strengthening and multiplying the number of T-defensive cells, increasing production of antibodies through the B-cells, and achieving dissolution of possible existing "immune blockages" through a reduction of too many T-control cells. Here as well, prostaglandin E1 is involved as an important immunoregulatory substance, which also protects the cell membranes and makes them more resistant against "attacks" from the outside, in addition to supporting the vital vesicular respiration. In the case of an intense and lasting damage to the inner respiration, the cells can become fermenting cells and the respiratory metabolism can become a fermentation metabolism. However, diminished vesicular respiration is not only a favorable breeding ground for bacteria and other pathogenic germs but can also lead to the occurrence of cancer.

The role of antioxidants for vesicular respiration should be mentioned once again, along with their role as catchers of free radicals, which have the effect of damaging tissue through attacks on the body's cells and are also involved in the occurrence of cancer, among other diseases. Apart from the components with antioxidant qualities in black cumin itself, such as thymoquinone, it is recommended that additional antioxidants be taken, such as those in the form of betacarotine (provitamin A) and tocopherol (vitamin E). Betacarotine and tocopherol, which are among the fat-soluble vitamins, protect the fat-containing cell membranes from attacks by the free radicals. Since unsaturated fatty acids are particularly quick to oxidate as a result of their substantial responsiveness, both the black cumin oil and the capsules usually have an additional dose of betacarotine and tocopherol added to protect against reactive oxygen.

Is It Possibly an Anticancer Drug?

Even if serious and complex clinical pictures like cancer could be treated exclusively through an intact immune system, black cumin oil certainly is not *the* new anticancer drug but can solely be understood to be a measure that supports the therapy. Incidentally, its comparable effect on "hardenings and old tumors" has been known since Pliny, which means for almost 2,000 years. Several years ago, laboratory experiments at a cancer research institute in South Carolina provided scientific proof that black cumin oil has not only a generally regulating effect on the immune system and increases the number of immune cells and antibodies but also:

- stimulates the formation of bone marrow cells
- protects the body cells from viruses
- destroys tumor cells
- increases the production of interferon

Through the intensified formation of the messenger substance *interferon*, a protein-like product of the cell metabolism in living cells that are infected with weakly pathogenic viruses, the growth of harmful microorganisms can be detectably inhibited. The American studies are based on the assumption that a strengthened and revitalized immune system can once again recognize and destroy tumor cells. The findings of comparable tests at the University of Alexandria (Egypt) in 1997 also confirm the inhibiting effect of *Nigella sativa*/black seed on tumor growth.

Despite these wonderful-sounding qualities, black cumin oil cannot "heal" but gives the sick person an effective instrument for self-help and personal responsibility for his or her body and health. However, its greatest advantage could exist in the perspective of not even permitting cancer to occur in the first place according to the motto that *prevention is better than healing* through the strengthening of an intact immune system and cleansing the body of cytotoxins. Using black cumin oil as a treatment for at least three months with the two main goals of strengthening the immune system and detoxifying the intestines is certainly not only an effective way of supporting any type of cancer therapy when there is existing disease, but also a good prophylaxis that prevents it from even breaking out in the first place. More detailed information on this is contained in the chapters "Recommendations for Oral Ingestion" and "Prevention."

Diabetes

Diabetes mellitus is among the wide-spread chronic diseases of our age. It is a serious dysfunction of the metabolism, based on a disturbed function of the pancreas and insufficient production of insulin. While juvenile diabetes, the type I diabetes that is usually congenital, shows an absolute insulin deficiency and therefore dependency on the administration of insulin, type II diabetes is characterized by a relative lack of insulin. A generally diminishing secretion of insulin, as well as a reduced ability of the cells to react to insulin, lead to an increase in the blood-sugar level. There are a number of contributing factors in the occurrence of type II diabetes, including an improper diet, an allergic predisposition, and stress because: when the blood "begins to boil," the blood-sugar level also rises, additional insulin must be produced and this places too much strain on the pancreas. This form of diabetes isn't necessarily dependent on insulin but can also be brought under control by losing weight, maintaining a certain diet, and taking specific active ingredients to stimulate the production of insulin.

A correlation between diabetes and essential fatty acids has been presumed for some time now. Insulin deficiency not only produces disturbances in the carbohydrate metabolism, but also in the fat metabolism, whereby unphysiologically high amounts of fatty acids result. These can lower the pH-value of the blood and lead to an acidemia of the blood with severe clouding of consciousness, up to a state of coma.

77

The damaging of the fat metabolism also causes intense arteriosclerotic changes of the vessels and high blood pressure.

More recent American research has now been able to prove a reduction of blood sugar through the ingestion of black cumin oil. This can presumably be explained through the prostaglandin synthesis since prostaglandin E1 has a hormone-like effect similar to that of insulin, as well as being able to intensify its effect in the metabolism. When black cumin is ingested, the blood-sugar value should be controlled by a doctor on a regular basis since it may drop so rapidly that an inadequate sugar level in the blood could occur.

As a welcome accompanying phenomenon, it was possible to determine that both the risk of vascular disease and pathological changes of the retina were reduced, as well as possible damage to the nervous function was improved.

The Hormonal System (Using the Example of PMS)

The female cycle is regulated by the female sexual hormones, meaning estrogen, progesteron, and prolactin, and their relationship to each other. Menstrual complaints are often connected with metabolic diseases since although a harmoniously functioning hormonal system is also associated with the immune system, the nervous system, and the psyche, the same also applies to a balanced metabolism.

The variety of complaints that can occur in the corpus-luteum phase of the menstrual cycle and are the most intense before the start of the period are summarized as "premenstrual syndrome" (PMS). This can include a feeling of tension in the breasts, swelling of the hands and legs, the formation of edema, abdominal cramps, migraines and muscle pain, as well as impure skin and very oily hair. Among the psychological symptoms that are often even more troublesome are extreme mood swings, intense irritability, difficulties in concentration, and an uneven temper, up to the point of depressive tendencies.

That PMS is primarily caused by neither psychological nor lasting endocrinal disorders is now considered as substantiated. However, numerous studies indicate that a metabolic disorder is the triggering factor. A well-balanced metabolism requires an adequate and harmonious supply of protein, carbohydrates, and fats. It has been possible to determine a deficiency or absorption disturbance of the essential fatty acids in women with PMS. As a result, an increased supply of them are necessary since the body's own conversion of them into prostaglandin E1 regulates the release of hormones, as well as causing an increase in the tonus of the smooth musculature in the sexual organs.

The positive effect of black cumin on menstruation that is too weak or painful, for fertility, pregnancy, and for lactation after the birth has traditionally been passed down in the folk medicine of the Near East, India, and also Europe. More recent studies have confirmed that modern women's diseases or those that have only been recognized in modern times such as the premenstrual syndrome and the complaints of menopause, in which at least a series of causes or triggers also interact, responded very positively to specific or even preventive treatment with black cumin oil.

Neurodermitis

Neurodermitis or *atopical eczema* is one of the great chronic diseases that have been considered incurable to a large extent up to now. An entire complex of causes is involved so that medical science doesn't really know what to do and speaks of a "multifactoral pathological process." In addition, neurodermitis manifests itself quite individually with a great variety of forms in those affected.

Neurodermitis is genetically caused, meaning it is congenital. It can, but does not always, already occur in infants and starts with cradle cap. There is quite frequently an allergic disposition as well, so that it can occur in connection with bronchial asthma and hay fever. On the other hand, it cannot be proved that clearly determined allergens are the sole cause but the increased flight of pollen, external toxins, certain foods and substances like alcohol and tobacco, as well as preservatives, can cause downright "attacks." Experts therefore like to also call it a "multiple allergy."

However, neurodermitis sometimes isn't defined as an allergy because it occurs with striking frequency in situations of radical change like puberty or menopause; hormonal factors, as well as undoubtedly psychological factors, play a role here. The *causes* and the *triggers* apparently must also be differentiated in neurodermitis.

How diversified such a clinical picture is can already be read in the medical literature describing the accompanying symptoms of skin diseases: the itch that is considered to be a complex occurrence "in which the pain-sensing organs, the vegetative system, histamines, inner secretion, and inner organs, the vascular system of the skin, the cortex of the brain, and the psyche participate."

Neurodermitis is also discussed in relation to food intolerances, causing a so-called "adaptation-exhaustion syndrome" of the immune system. This means: through the combination of certain foods that can usually be tolerated quite well, exaggerated allergic reactions occur in the form of the above-mentioned attacks on the basis of pollen, alcohol, physical exertion, or psychological strain.

In addition to the allergic disposition, an abnormal metabolism of the essential fatty acids and the prostaglandins through enzyme deficiency is considered to be proved. An inhibition in the release of prostaglandin E1, for example, can cause a disturbance of the cellular and humoral immune systems and an increased tendency towards inflammations, etc. An improvement of the symptoms can be supported by an increased intake of essential fatty acids as a food supplement (10-15% of the overall supply of calories). Black cumin oil also offers the possibility of an *external* treatment, which not only relieves the itching but also has an anti-inflammatory effect and speeds up the healing process.

Moreover, there is a close relationship between skin eczema, certain intestinal bacteria, and yeast fungi or molds. A lack of lactobacillus (*Lactobacillus acidophilus*), above all, can almost always be found in neurodermitis patients, for example. These have the task of lowering the pH-value in the intestines and suppressing putrefactive bacterium. A special factor of danger for neurodermitis is the yeast fungus *Candida albicans*, which, when it receives the opportunity of multiplying too intensely, releases metabolic toxins typical for fungi. The immune system reacts with exaggerated reactions, so to speak, to an "allergen" that has actually settled within the intestines. In this situation, the black cumin oil treatment can be highly recommended in particular for thorough intestinal detoxification as a supplement to an intestinal therapy through symbiostic management with useful strains of bacteria. Further information on this can be found in the following chapters on "Recommendations for Oral Ingestion" and "Prevention."

A Necessary Chapter:
Possible Therapy Restrictions

The statement that taking black cumin oil is connected with no "risks and side-effects" can only be made under certain restrictions:

There must be no doubt that it is a first-class quality of black cumin oil, which means: natural cultivation that has been personally supervised, if possible, with seeds of a non-toxic sort, guaranteed cold-pressing without solvents, and the greatest possible protection against oxidation in the further processing steps, in transportation, and in storage. As far as possible, attention should therefore be paid to certain quality features when buying black cumin oil. "Side-effects" in the gastrointestinal tract, as well as damage to the kidney function, can occur particularly through oxidation. Because of the alkaloid and saponin content, an exact observation of the individual reaction is also advisable since we can hardly expect a medicinal plant to be both highly effective and completely harmless at the same time. The old advice given by Paracelsus—that whether a medicinal plant has the effect of a medicine or of a poison depends on the dosage—applies here, just as it does in so many other cases!

The trade should also be sure there is proof on the grower's or producer's certificates or have these provided by another source. They not only give information about the peroxide value and possible residue but also on the composition of the fatty acids. It has been determined that the effectiveness of oils that have been mixed may be restricted up to 50% when used for therapeutic treatment and as a remedy for prevention. This is why it is important to pay attention to the statement of whether there is 100% *pure black cumin oil.*

When ingesting black cumin oil, it should also be taken into consideration that the prostaglandin synthesis in the body occurs very slowly and that the supply of unsaturated fatty acids must therefore take place on a regular basis and over a longer period of time, at least three and sometimes even up to six months. However, if the condition does *not* improve even after taking black cumin oil for a longer period of time, a metabolism that is inadequately stimulated by enzymes, and therefore a deficient process of transforming the essential fatty acids in the tissue hormones, could be the cause. A disturbed or acidotic intestinal milieu then exists so that the enzyme process is disrupted and, above all, a deficiency of delta-6-desaturase occurs. Improper diet, allergens, psychological strain, and aging processes are seen to be the main causes for this disorder. Through the acidosis of the organism an increased consumption of mineral substances often arises, which can then easily lead to deficiency symptoms. In addition to a complete change of lifestyle, an increased supply of vitamins (B and C) can also help, available in such fruits as papayas, pineapples, and mangos. These are said to have a high level of enzyme mobility. Food supplementation through trace elements is also recommended, especially zinc—and, above all, much patience!

Even with the precondition of having a black cumin oil showing first-class quality features, ingestion may result in an—usually temporary—overreaction of the gastrointestinal tract. This can possibly be explained through a vehement reaction of the intestinal fungi and the corresponding detoxification symptoms, which accompany the cleansing and purification from toxic substances and harmful microorganisms. An overly sensitive gastrointestinal tract, as well as secondary allergies in the form of food intolerance, may also be possible causes. As the reports on personal experiences prove, intensive detoxification symptoms may be observed that are not in the gastrointestinal tract but affect the skin and can additionally be expressed in extreme fatigue and exhaustion. For all these symptoms, it is very important to drink a great deal of spring water and herbal teas for the elimination of foreign substances. If necessary, the dosage can be strongly reduced or discontinued for a time in order to leave enough time for the inner reprogramming of not only the immune system but also the entire organism.

The Right Dosage and Further Recommendations for Oral Ingestion

Black cumin can be used internally and externally in the form of seeds, as pure oil or oil processed into gelatine capsules, and as essential oil. The ground or powdered seeds are both a healthy and tasty enrichment for the kitchen. They can also be used in tea mixtures, for inhalation, and for skin packs. The oil has a concentrated effect for curative purposes; in addition, it is already taken in by the mucous membrane of the mouth and can be directly absorbed by the small intestine. The oil is also offered in the form of gelatine capsules; each capsule contains, according to the manufacturer, 400 – 500 mg of black cumin oil, which is normally enriched with natural vitamin E (D-alpha-tocopherol) as an antioxidant. That it is offered in capsules may perhaps be related to the somewhat unaccustomed acrid taste of some types of oils, but consumer habits are certain to also play a role here: the oil is not always practical to take at work or even at a restaurant, children don't like the pure oil, and "liver types" may possibly not tolerate it. However, the processing of black cumin oil into capsules is reflected not only in a distinctly higher price but also slows down absorption in the body. It also raises the question of the "kosher" origins of the colloidal substance of the gelatine, which comes from an animal source. The use of vegetable or vegan capsules is not possible in the manufacture of black cumin oil capsules since these would dissolve.

The use of black cumin is compatible with every other type of medical treatment. However, it should be clear from the start that this is a natural and comparatively gentle remedy and no immediate healing of acute symptoms should be expected. Apart from digestive complaints, just taking the oil every once in a while can hardly be helpful. Chronic complaints in particular require taking the oil on a longer term and more regular basis in the form of a treatment that should last from at least three months to even six months. Because of the origin of black cumin, the recommendation to take it during the warm seasons instead of the cold seasons seems to make sense.

Three plans for taking black cumin oil:

❀ *The simplest method*
3 x daily 1/2 – 1 teaspoon of oil or 1 – 2 capsules shortly before or during the 3 main meals

❀ *The stepwise method*
at the beginning, for 2 – 3 weeks 3 x daily 1 teaspoon of oil (corresponds to approx. 25 drops) or 6 – 8 capsules à 500 mg at mealtimes; as a maintenance dosage and for prevention 3 – 4 capsules daily or 3 – 4 x daily 1/2 teaspoon of oil

❀ *The bread method*
3 x daily 25 drops, also before the meals, dripped onto a little piece of whole-grain bread. Chew well and soak with saliva before swallowing (has the advantage of stimulating the formation of enzymes in the saliva)

❀ **Reduced dosage for children:**
3 weeks 2 x daily 1/2 teaspoon or 1 capsule; then 1 – 2 capsules daily.

❀ **Contraindictions**
It is generally not advisable to ingest black cumin preparations during pregnancy since the tissue hormones (prostaglandins) formed within the body from it can cause a dialation of the cervix and possibly can trigger premature labor as a result.

Further Observations and Recommendations

❀ Although general guidelines can be specified for the dosage, they are still based on individual experience. Black cumin oil of a medically pure quality usually cannot only be taken over a longer period of time without risk, the dosage can also be increased for acute complaints (such as a pollen allergy) for a short time.

- At the beginning an occasional belching may occur, although this happens seldom, because of the digestant effect. This usually goes away on its own after a few days.

- When the gastrointestinal tract is particularly sensitive or a food allergy occurs now and then, it is better to start with a minimal dosage since vehement reactions may otherwise occur.

- Experience has shown that black cumin has a strongly cleansing effect and promotes all types of excretions, including those that occur through the skin as our largest "excretory organ." If the detoxification symptoms that have already been mentioned above occur while taking it on a regular basis, it is best to experiment a bit with the appropriate dosage so that you do not feel too unwell and, above all, remember to drink enough in order to wash out the toxins.

- If you eat the pure seeds, a slight irritation of the mucous membranes of the mouth and esophagus may occur for a short time. If the seeds are soaked in hot water, such as in a tea or for an inhalation, this effect does not occur.

- When using the seeds, be sure that you always crush or grind them *fresh* yourself when a fine powder is required for certain applications. For this reason, a ready-made black cumin shouldn't be purchased for either skin-care or use in the kitchen since the fact that it has lost some of its aroma or has a strikingly acrid taste is most likely an indication of oxidation.

- The ingestion of the essential oil is not recommended. Use it externally only in a diluted form since it is slightly irritating for the skin.

Prevention Is Better Than Healing

Black Cumin as a Preventive Treatment for the Immune System and for Intestinal Detoxification

Two very important possibilities for using black cumin, the regulation of the immune system and the cleansing and eliminatory effect on the digestive system (particularly the detoxification of the intestines) have already been mentioned a number of times. Both of these applications belong to the large area of *prevention* and *health care* and have a greater effect on the origins and possible causes of diseases than on symptoms that have already become manifest.

Black cumin's diverse modes of action on the *immune system* can be summarized under the general term of "harmonization." This means that a weakened defensive system is strengthened and can better protect itself from a great variety of pathogenic agents (germs); in the same manner, an immune system that shows an exaggerated reaction to irritating substances is regulated, leading to a relief of the allergic symptoms. Using the black cumin oil as a preventive treatment for a *prophylactic* effect can work wonders here, especially when it respectively takes place before the time period with the presumably greatest amount of stress: for the strengthening of the body's defenses against infections and diseases of the respiratory tract before the cold seasons and for the regulation of the immune system against allergic reactions in the spring before the flight of pollen. Such a preventive treatment with black cumin oil should last at least six weeks or even three months. For the initial six-week phase, a dose of 1/2 to 1 teaspoon of black cumin oil or 1 – 2 capsules are recommended 3 times a day. When a certain stabilization of the immune system has been achieved, the dose can be reduced by half and later continue as a "maintenance dose" through the use of black cumin together with food.

Intestinal detoxification is an important topic since intestinal toxins may have very grave consequences, as the saying by Paracelsus proves quite drastically—"death is found in the intestines." They are usually produced by harmful intestinal bacteria and yeast fungi, which can multiply too intensely and spread through the acidosis of the organism and a weakened defensive situation. As a result of fermentation processes, metabolic toxins are released and cannot be eliminated from the intestines primarily because of a tendency towards constipation that occurs at the same time.

These intestinal toxins can produce diverse symptoms of disease and lead up to functional damage of the organs. This includes much more than just the digestive complaints occurring at the beginning, the alternation between diarrhea and constipation, local inflammation of the bowels and flatulence, as well as symptoms such as inexplicable tiredness, states of fatigue, and chronic headache but also later, and above all with increasing age, vascular deposits (with the danger of vascular occlusion), chronic rheumatic complaints and arthritis, skin diseases, and allergic symptoms. For example, the yeast fungus *Candida albicans* is considered to be decidedly "useful" for promoting attacks of neurodermitis since the constant presence of a foreign substance living within the body can accordingly provoke exaggerated allergic defensive reactions of the immune system.

In the case of serious fungus diseases, black cumin can certainly just be used as a support and accompanying therapy for such measures as a special anti-fungal diet (no acid-forming foods, no sugar and white flour), fasting cures, and symbiotic management. The application of black cumin oil as a preventive treatment, which accompanies the strengthening of the immune system, is both less problematic and more promising of success. During the first weeks, take 1 teaspoon of black cumin oil with the three main meals or use the method of dripping about 25 drops on a small piece of whole-grain bread and chewing it well in order to stimulate the formation of enzymes in the saliva. After about 4 – 6 weeks, the ingestion can be limited to the main meal of the day.

Although black cumin has an extremely diverse range of applications, the regulation of the immune system and the detoxification of the intestines are foremost since these areas can be the starting point for many health disorders and the more serious diseases that develop as a result. In this process, the essential fatty acids mainly take over the function of immunoregulatory substances through the prostaglandins while the bitter principles and saponins (nigellin and melanthin) effect the digestive tract and intestinal cleansing in particular. As a complex remedy, black cumin once again obviously develops its merits here through the synergetic interaction of components that supplement each other in an excellent way.

Even in a purely preventive application of black cumin oil, the possible therapy restrictions and, in certain cases, also the recommendations for ingestion based on individual experiences, which have been compiled in the two previous chapters, should be observed.

Rinsing the Mouth with Black cumin Oil

Rinsing the mouth with sunflower oil is an old Russian folk remedy for activating the powers of self-healing, which essentially serves to basically detoxify the body. The Russian medical doctor F. Karach reintroduced this practice on the occasion of a convention of the Pan-Ukrainian Association of Oncologists and Bacteriologists. It has a beneficial effect on headaches, toothaches, bronchitis, eczemas, gastric and intestinal complaints, heart and kidney problems, chronic blood diseases, thrombosis, degenerative arthrosis, and women's diseases.

If the sunflower oil is completely or partially replaced by black cumin oil, the healing process can be even further supported by the latter's special qualities.

Renate Spannagel has passed on the following experiences: "Sunflower oil and 100% black cumin oil—a minimum of one teaspoon, maximum of one tablespoon—is to be leisurely swished back and forth in the mouth and sucked through the teeth for 15 to 20 minutes. At first it is syrupy, but then becomes increasingly thinner, after which it must be spit out. By no means should the oil be swallowed! The liquid that is spit out should be as white as milk. If it still is yellow, this is a sign that the rinsing wasn't done long enough.

After the oil is spit out, the teeth must be thoroughly cleaned and the mouth rinsed out with water a number of times. Then you should disinfect the oral cavity with warm water that has had a few drops of 100% pure tea tree oil added to it.

A great amount of bacteria, various germs, and other harmful substances can be found in the liquid that has been spit out. It is especially important to emphasize that the organism is increasingly detoxified during the sucking and swishing and a lastingly stabilized state of health can be achieved in this way. One of the most conspicuous effects of this method is that loose teeth become more firm and gum-bleeding is prevented. This effect is particularly intensified by the black cumin oil, which also normalizes an exaggerated sensation of hot and cold.

The best time to do this rinsing is in the morning before breakfast. In order to accelerate the healing process, the method can be repeated three times a day before meals. There is a possibility that an apparent worsening of the state of health occurs at the start. This feeling mainly comes about when the individual seats of disease begin to vanish. The treatment must be continued until the original strength, freshness, and peaceful sleep have once again been restored to the organism.

"Your Food Should Be Healing Remedies"

The exhortation with the complete wording, uttered by the famous Greek physician Hippocrates:

Your food should be healing remedies,
and your healing remedies should be food

is just as valid today as it was 2,500 years ago when it was first stated. The black cumin plant and the oil contained in its seeds fulfill this exhortation in a convincing manner.

The healing power of vegetable oils have been known to humanity since time immemorial. About at the same time as Hippocrates, the philosopher Democritus revealed the secret of his health up into ripe old age: "Honey inside, and oil outside!" This naturally refers above all to the olive oil, which was extracted either through cold first-pressing or the old impact method and also used for the preparation of foods. However, with the currently prevalent cultivation methods and oil-processing procedures, the restriction must be made that only naturally grown, cold-pressed, and chemically unadulterated oil earns the rating as a "food and healing remedy"—and this does not apply to refined oils or hardened fats.

In the industrial manufacturing and hardening of vegetable fats (like margarine), the chemical composition of the fatty acids changes into trans-fats or so-called "fatty acid cripples." Although these are built into the cell walls in the metabolism, they can no longer fulfill their actual function. The cell walls become more permeable, which leads to the increased formation of free radicals and pathological changes of the metabolism, also including an increase of the cholesterol level. Cholesterol is a building block for the cell walls and the nerve tissue. As a precursor to the bile acids and in the role of a vital hormone, it has a decisive task within the body. However, cholesterol that has been changed and exists in excess amounts can deposit itself on the inner walls of the vessels and constrict them. This can be the beginning of an arteriosclerosis, which often has life-threatening effects.

The causes of a cholesterol level that is too elevated is, among other things, attributed to eating too much fat with a high content of saturated fatty acids from animal sources.

Particularly important within this context and in general for the activation of the metabolism are vegetable fats and oils with primarily unsaturated fatty acids. Their chemical compounds form the preconditions for an impecable burning of protein and fat and thereby inhibit the depositing of excess fats as "fatty tissue." A diet with too many calories, particularly a high level of fat consumption with mainly saturated fatty acids and the overweight that often results from this are among the well-known risk factors for an elevated cholesterol level, cardiovascular diseases, as well as diabetes and gout.

Nutritionist have pointed out that a complete omittance of fat does not lead to weight loss but that a conscious supply of about 20 grams of native cold-pressed vegetable oils with unsaturated fatty acids in particular supports the necessary burning process. It has also been discovered that unsaturated fatty acids, and above all the essential fatty acids (primarily linoleic and linolenic acids) are vital for the regulation of important bodily functions. Although earlier laboratory tests determined that an portion of 1% of the entire calorie consumption in the form of essential fatty acids is necessary to promote normal growth and healthy development, today prominent sources once again repeatedly recommend increasing the calorie supply in the form of essential fatty acids to 10% – 15%. In the meantime, it has been proved that such a high dosage shows an extremely desirable effect in numerous diseases and certainly for their prevention as well.

Pure cold-pressed vegetable oils are therefore important components of a diet of natural food. Since their chemical structure changes in a way detrimental to health through intensive heating, it is best to enjoy them with raw vegetable salads. In this form—in small amounts and perhaps together with a neutral-tasting oil—the very aromatic black cumin oil can also be used, whereby 2 grams = 1 teaspoon of oil are adequate per day as a food supplement. Of course, it can also be used for the preparation of vegetable and meat dishes, to which it lends an "Oriental" touch, but should not be cooked or fried along with them. If possible, sprinkle it quite sparingly on the food right before the cooking time is over.

The use of black cumin seed as a spice in cooking and, above all, in baking, has been traditionally handed down. The foods become more tasty with it and more easily digestible at the same time because of its digestant effect. In earlier times, the seeds used to serve as a substitute for pepper or were used like coriander. Since they have a spicy, hot, and sometimes perhaps even a acrid or bitter taste for some people, it probably is not everyone's cup of tea to use larger amounts of them so that the curative effect becomes secondary to that of a spicy food supplement.

Black cumin seeds can be sprinkled raw on salads (like ground pepper) or added to vegetables, or they can also be roasted beforehand in an iron pan without the use of fat. In addition, they can be finely ground (in a coffee mill) or somewhat more coarsely crushed in a mortar for putting them into a bread dough or sprinkling them like poppy and sesame onto flat breads and baked goods. There are no limits to an individual's imagination and intuition here. However, some recipe suggestions have been compiled at the close of this book.

Black cumin seeds can also be used for tea infusions, either pure or in various herbal tea mixtures, which serve both to improve the taste and also provide a more specific use against certain complaints. Because of the sensitive components, an infusion of the seeds should be made with hot but not boiling water (about 80°C), just like green tea is prepared. According to the selection of the other ingredients, they have a very good curative effect for digestive problems, colds, or sleep disturbances, for example. Various tea recipes have been included in the following chapter under the respective clinical pictures. Since sometimes neither doing a preventive treatment nor reaching into the spice rack helps, this is called:

THERAPEUTIC APPLICATIONS* AND SPECIAL SELECTED RECIPES

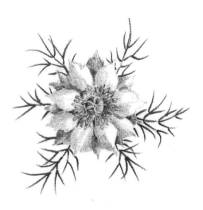

*The symptoms and clinical pictures are treated in larger groups that have an inner relation here instead of in alphabetical order. In as far as they were available, personal experiences and short case histories have been documented.

General Lowered Resistance

Through a disturbance of the immune system a generalized state of lowered resistance can occur. This initially expresses itself in vegetative nervous exhaustion, a greater suscepti- bility to infections, the tendency towards chronically repeat- ing complaints or illnesses and can ultimately become a breeding ground for malignant dysfunctions. Because of its polyunsaturated fatty acids and the added antioxidant vita- mins, black cumin oil is effective and contributes to the strengthening and revitalization of the immune system when used over a longer period of time as a preventive treatment. Enzymes should be supplied to the body as well.

RECOMMENDATIONS FOR USE:

* *Inhalation* for general stimulation and activation of the immune system: Add 1 cup of freshly ground black cu- min seeds, or 1/2 tablespoon of fatty oil, or 5 drops of essential oil to 1 liter of hot water and inhale the steam for 10 – 15 minutes.
* *Bath*: Add 5 – 8 drops of essential black cumin oil, emul- sified with some cream, to the bath water.
* *Massage*: Mix 100 ml jojoba oil or macadamia nut oil with 15 – 20 drops of essential black cumin oil and use for a whole-body massage.
* *Internally* for the stabilization of the immune system by way of a longer preventive course of treatment: daily 2 – 3 times 1/2 – 1 teaspoon of black cumin oil or 2 – 3 cap- sules at the main meals for a period of 3 weeks; after- wards, daily 1 teaspoon of black cumin oil or 2 – 3 cap- sules with one main meal for a period of about 4 – 6 months.

Further information on immune-system preventive treatment with black cumin oil can be found in the chapter "Prevention Is Better Than Healing."

General Lowered Resistance
with Vegetative Exhaustion

This frequently occurs when a person experiences negative stress and the permanent feeling of being overstrained. A treatment with black cumin oil has a strengthening effect and leads to a significant improvement in performance.

RECOMMENDATION FOR USE:

❀ Drink a mixture of one glass of freshly squeezed orange juice (vitamin C) or carrot juice (vitamin A) with one teaspoon of black cumin oil and one teaspoon of honey twice a day. In addition, three black cumin oil capsules a day can be taken, for the maximum length of one month.

The suggestions for external use under "General Lowered Resistance" are very suitable as a supplementary measure.

Potency Disorders as an Expression
of General Weakness

The people of the Orient have long known what is good for potency disorders, meaning intermittently occurring impotence (medically paraphrased as an "erectile dysfunction"). Black cumin is among the time-tested home remedies for strengthening the male libido. It has the effect of dilating the blood vessels and therefore supporting the circulation, stimulating bodily secretions, and promoting an increased release of the masculine sexual hormone. In addition, it also has a gentle psychological effect against feelings of ill-humor.

The medicine of the Orient prefers to mix black cumin with other potency-increasing remedies. Here are two traditional recipes that have been handed down:

❀ Boil one tablespoon (approx. 5 grams) of fenugreek seeds (*Trigonella foenum-graecum*) in one cup of water, let the liquid cool off and then strain. Drink mixed with one teaspoon each of honey and black cumin oil in the evening. If available, also mix in 1/2 grams of ambergris.

✺ Mix one cup (approx. 100 grams) of finely ground black cumin seeds with one cup of true elecampane (*Inula helenium*), two tablespoons of fenugreek, and one tablespoon of oregano. Take one tablespoon a day together with some honey.

Lowered Resistance with Auto-Aggressive Immune Reaction—Allergic and Rheumatic Symptoms

The other extreme of a disturbed bodily defense is an excessive immune reaction, which can cause allergies and various rheumatic diseases, as well as serious chronic illnesses like leukemia and multiple sclerosis. Here as well, a preventive treatment using black cumin oil is recommended for a gentle but thorough change of condition.

RECOMMENDATIONS FOR APPLICATION:

✺ 3 x daily, one teaspoon of black cumin oil with each of the three main meals for the length of three weeks. Afterwards, continue to take one teaspoon of black cumin oil or 2 – 3 capsules with a main meal daily for the length of 4 – 6 months.

Ms. Gerry R., 55 years old, had suffered from lympathic leukemia for eight months. This had been preceded by an autoimmune illness. In addition, she had suffered for about one year from a painful arthritis of the right hip joint so that she could no longer rest on this side of the body and it was impossible for her to walk a longer distance.

The medically supervised treatment began with a careful dosage of 3 x one capsule on the first two days; it was then increased to 3 x two capsules a day, and one teaspoon of black cumin oil was taken additionally 2 x a day.

At the beginning, the patient stated that there were reactions like flatulence and belching. However, these diminished after about the first two weeks. In addition, frequent headaches and an increasing tiredness occurred during this time period, which could probably be ascribed to the beginning elimination of toxic substances.

After about two months, the complaints in the hip joint subsided. The patient could once again lie on the afflicted side with almost no pain, and she was also once again able to cover longer distances on foot. In addition, her sleep improved.

After a period of almost three months, the laboratory values were checked. In comparison to the preliminary examination that had taken place before the start of the black cumin treatment, an actual improvement could be determined in some of the disease-related laboratory values (such as the leucocyte count and the IgG). Other results had remained unchanged, yet no deterioration had occurred anywhere.

Ms. R. continued taking two black cumin oil capsules 3 x daily as a maintenance dose.

Inflammatory and Allergic Skin Diseases (Dermatitis and Eczemas)

These include skin rashes that are connected with intensive itching, allergic skin inflammations and edemas, nettle rash, eczema, and neurodermitis. Through the combination of its components, black cumin has an effect that is simultaneously anti-inflammatory and immunoregulatory. It can be applied very well both internally and externally for:

- Elimination of itching
- Harmonization of overreactive immune system
- Support of complete healing for afflicted skin areas.

Since a long tradition exists for this form of application, some of the old recipes have been included here.

ANCIENT COPTIC RECIPE AGAINST ITCHING OF THE SKIN (SCABIES):

Pulverize the black cumin seeds and bring to a boil together with garlic, sodium carbonate, ripened vinegar (apple-cider vinegar is also good for this purpose), fir resin, and radish oil. After it has cooled down, use as an ointment. The prognosis: "The afflicted skin will peel off. Rinse with warm water after three days."

AYURVEDIC RECIPE AGAINST ECZEMA AND PSORIASIS:

Two ounces each of finely ground black cumin seeds, *Psoralea corylifolia*, *Bdellium* (balsam tree), and one ounce of sulphur is worked into a paste with coconut oil and applied to the affected parts of the skin.

The use of black cumin and apple-cider vinegar against skin rashes has been handed down ever since the time of Pliny (1st century):

❀ Grind black cumin seeds and mix with apple-cider vinegar, then apply like a plaster

❀ Is also mentioned by Hieronymus Bock (16th century) as a remedy "against tubers, tumors, skin herpes, and acute injuries"

❀ Mixed with urine (!), it also helps against warts and thorn warts (according to Tabernaemontanus, 18th century)

❀ *Black cumin skin oil against eczema:*
Heat 3 tablespoons of black cumin oil in a pan and fry 3 tablespoons of finely ground black cumin seeds in it. Strain and let cool. Store in a cool place and apply cold—this gives it a stronger relieving effect.

OLD ARABIAN RECIPE AGAINST ECZEMA:

Externally:

❀ Black cumin paste: Boil 2 parts apple-cider vinegar and 1 part ground black cumin seeds and work into a paste by adding 1 part starch or some other thickening agent. After this mixture has cooled, apply several times daily to the affected areas of the skin. Healing earth can also be used in place of the starch or in addition to it.

❀ *Black cumin tincture:* Mix together 2 parts apple-cider vinegar and 1 part ground black cumin seeds and leave to stand for 6 hours. Strain and let stand for another 24 hours. Drain off the excess liquid and mix the residue that has been deposited with black cumin oil in a ratio of 1:1. Apply several times a day.

❀ *Variation:* The residue is mixed with healing earth and apple-cider vinegar in a ratio of 4:2:1. Heat while stirring for 2 – 3 minutes. Before applying to the skin (the best method is over night), mix with black cumin oil in a ratio of 1:1.

Internally for support:

❀ Boil 1 part finely ground black cumin seeds in 2 parts apple-cider vinegar. While stirring this, slowly add 1 part black cumin oil. Let cool off and put in a cool place. Take 1 teaspoon of this 3 x daily.

TREATMENT SUGGESTIONS FOR CHRONIC ALLERGIC DERMATITIS:

❀ *Externally:* Rub the affected skin areas with undiluted black cumin oil or black cumin oil mixed with tea tree oil in a ratio of 1:1; immediate excellent effect against itching but first try out on a small spot of the skin to avoid counter-reactions. In some cases, a mixture using essential lavender or chamomile oil is also recommended.

❀ *Facial steam baths:* Put 1 – 2 tablespoons of black cumin seeds, or 1/2 tablespoon of fatty oil, or 5 drops of essential oil in 1 liter of hot water and allow the steam to take effect on the facial skin at least once a day for 10 – 15 minutes.

❀ *Internally* (longer-term application as preventive treatment): 3 times daily 1 teaspoon of black cumin oil or 2 – 3 capsules with the 3 main meals; also continue after the acute complaints subside as a maintenance dose with one meal a day.

A young man, who works as an auto mechanic, suffered from a chronic allergic dermatitis (possibly an allergic contact eczema). It primarily appeared on his hands, which became reddened and extremely swollen, and certainly hindered him extensively in his work. In addition, there were frequently deep fissures with bleeding.

After three weeks of taking 2 – 3 teaspoon of black cumin oil every day and applying a black cumin cream at the same time, a slow normalization of the skin cells could be observed. The massive symptoms in the form of bleeding and cracked skin disappeared first, and then the swelling and reddening of the hands gradually subsided as well.

Dirk S., 28 years old, had an allergic spot on his right temple that was about the size of a silver dollar. It appeared about once a week. The man had used a cortisone ointment for three years, but because of unexplained causes the allergic symptom returned time and again.

He began a treatment with black cumin oil and not only rubbed the affected skin spot with it, but also supported the treatment with the internal ingestion of 2 – 3 capsules 3 x daily. After just three weeks, the ugly spot had disappeared permanently.

Special Case: Neurodermitis

Neurodermitis is a chronic inflammatory skin disease that primarily occurs in the bends of the joints, on the arms, on the throat, neck, shoulders, and chest, as well as on the face. The formation of eczema is often accompanied by tormenting itching, swelling, and scaling. Why this disease has grown at such a drastic rate, and increasingly already particularly in children, has not yet been clarified. Neurodermitis is attributed to the combined influence of several factors, including allergies, and manifests itself in individuals with greatly differing forms.

Because of its immunoregulating and anti-inflammatory qualities, black cumin at least can cause a strong relief of the symptoms or even lead to their complete absence.

INGESTION RECOMMENDATION

- ❀ (only as a longer-term preventive treatment and in most cases as support for other therapies): 1 teaspoon of black cumin oil or 2 capsules 2 – 3 times daily with the main meals.
- ❀ *Externally* (to reduce the itching and for quicker healing): Mix black cumin oil in a ratio of 1:1 with tea tree oil and dab onto the affected skin areas several times a day. Or mix 100 ml jojoba oil with 20 ml black cumin oil and 20 drops of tea tree oil and carefully rub into the skin.

It is important that you use this application cautiously and do a sensitivity test beforehand!

Mycosis

A weakened immune system also contributes to the infection of the organism with harmful fungi. A further factor is an improper diet (rich in sugar but low in roughage and the resulting acidosis as the ideal terrain for pathogenic germs. Fungi prefer to settle in the intestines, in the vagina, and on the skin. They can be treated with black cumin oil because of its immune-strengthening effect, as well as its anti-mycotic qualities, in a way that at least is supportive of the therapy.

Skin fungi

OLD ARABIAN RECIPE FOR SKIN FUNGI

This requires 1 glass each of apple-cider vinegar, finely ground black cumin seeds, and black cumin oil. Boil the vinegar and add the black cumin to it. Strain the mixture and then add the oil. Mix everything together well and apply to the affected spots several times a day.

Modern tips:
* ❀ Starch or healing earth can be used in place of the oil to bind if a more solid consistency is desired.
* ❀ First let the mixture cool off before adding the oil and then store in the refrigerator!
* ❀ The affected skin areas can also be treated with pure black cumin oil or mixed with tea tree oil in a ratio of 1:1.

Intestinal fungi

INTERNAL APPLICATION FOR THE DETOXIFICATION OF INTESTINAL FUNGI

The guidelines on the course of preventive-treatment application for intestinal detoxification, as described in detail in the chapter on "Prevention Is Better Than Healing," apply here.

❀ Daily 1 teaspoon or 6 capsules of black cumin oil 3 x daily with the meals for 3 weeks; then reduce to 3 capsules.

OLD ARABIAN RECIPE AGAINST INTESTINAL FUNGI

❀ Boil 1 glass of apple-cider vinegar, 1/2 glass of finely ground black cumin seeds and 1/2 glass of black cumin oil to a syrupy consistency. Take 1 teaspoon before meals 3 x a day.

VAGINAL FUNGI

As an accompanying measure for the intestinal detoxification, a local therapy with *essential* black cumin oil can also be tried as follows:

❀ Clean the vaginal area with highly diluted essential oil (5 drops to 1 liter of water) or take a hip bath in it.

❀ To make an "aromatic tampon," mix 10 drops of essential black cumin oil with 30 ml of jojoba oil. Soak the tampon in this mixture and then insert it. Change a number of times a day.

Allergic and Infectious Disorders
of the Respiratory System

This usually includes allergically caused bronchial asthma, pollen allergy (hay fever), chronic bronchitis, pulmonary emphysema, stubborn hacking cough, and virus infections in the form of a cold that manifest themselves in symptoms like a runny nose, coughing, sinusitis, etc.

Because of its essential active ingredients nigellone and thymoquinone, as well as the prostaglandins, black cumin has a secretion-dissolving and vasodilating effect. This means that it is strongly relaxing for the respiratory system. Supported by the regulating influence on the immune system, complaints in this area of application have an extraordinarily positive response to a black cumin treatment in almost every case. However, for diseases like severe asthma, note that it is absolutely restricted to the role of *supporting the therapy*!

Everywhere, in the Near East and Middle East, and in all parts of Europe, the following method has been handed down since time immemorial—perhaps because it is so astoundingly simple and highly effective at the same time:

INHALATION FOR ASTHMA AND HAY FEVER

❀ Put 1 glass of fresh, finely ground black cumin seeds in a bowl and infuse with 1 liter of boiling water. Inhale the steam for about 15 minutes.

Further tips:
❀ Especially effective in the evening before going to bed
❀ Use 1/2 tablespoon of fatty oil or 5 drops of essential oil in place of or in addition to the seeds
❀ Don't use boiling water—just hot water with a temperature of about 80°C
❀ Cover your head with a large towel
❀ Also use for pollen allergy (hay fever)

❀ Additionally rub black cumin oil onto the chest—use the fatty oil undiluted or mix a few drops of essential black cumin oil and tea tree oil with a non-irritating body oil.

OLD EUROPEAN RECIPE FOR A TINCTURE (is mentioned in the various herbals of the 16th to 18th centuries)

❀ Crush black cumin seeds and simmer in wine, then strain. Drinking a warm glass of this in the morning and evening "warms and cleanses the chest and lungs, softens the thick, viscous mucous, relieves the sputum, helps when there is shortness of breath and wheezing."

OLD ARABIAN RECIPE FOR A SYRUP

❀ 1 part ground black cumin seeds
2 parts honey
1 crushed clove of garlic or the corresponding amount of grated ginger

Mix well with each other. Take 1 teaspoon of this syrup every morning for several weeks.

❀ Garlic/ginger and honey can also be used together with the black cumin seeds for the inhalation described above.

OLD (STILL VERY RECOMMENDABLE) TEA RECIPE

❀ 3 parts black cumin seeds
2 parts liquorice root
1 part anise seed

Crush finely and infuse with hot water. Let draw for 10 minutes, filter, and drink sweetened with honey. Has a good effect on the stomach at the same time and is very relaxing.

In addition to the inhalation that has already been described, a longer period of taking the black cumin oil as a preventive measure for regulating the immune system is recommended. If possible, this should be started several months before the pollen begins its flight and continued into the summer.

❀ For prevention: take 1/2 – 1 teaspoon of black cumin oil or 1 – 2 capsules 2 – 3 times a day

❀ As highest dosage during the time of pollen flight: 1 – (maximum) 2 teaspoons or 2 -3 capsules 2 – 3 x daily.

Flus and Colds

As protection against a general susceptibility to infections and for prevention purposes in particular, a longer-term preventive black cumin oil treatment is recommended. Influenza infections should at least occur less frequently. When the typical symptoms of a cold occur despite this, black cumin also has a great deal to offer as first aid from the home medicine cabinet. A great number of internal and external application possibilities have already been recommended in the old European sources—probably because of the cold and wet weather. The inhalation already described under "Asthma and Hay Fever" is very popular. The following remedies are also useful against runny nose, catarrh, and breathing difficulties:

❀ Burn black cumin seeds on charcoals (today we can naturally use the essential oil in a fragrance lamp as well)
❀ Crush black cumin seeds, tie into a little silk or linen cloth and smell it frequently
❀ Roast black cumin and anise seeds in an iron pan, moisten with distilled marjoram water, tie into a little cloth, and smell it frequently

OLD TIME-TESTED RECIPE FOR NOSE DROPS

Today we can make it easy on ourselves and rub the entire nasal area, including the nostrils, with black cumin oil when we have colds with intensive sinusitis. This also has a expectorant effect when inhaled. The two following special recipes, handed down from the 18th century, also help in cases of *sinusitis and chronic suppurative catarrh of the frontal sinuses.*

❀ Mix crushed black cumin seeds with old tree oil (meaning olive oil). Lean the head back as far as possible and drip 3 – 4 drops into each nostril.

Very good tip: fill the mouth with water so that the oil cannot flow into it.

For advanced users

❀ Crush nard seeds (black cumin) together with orris-root (*Iris florentina*) and sieve to make a fine powder. Simmer equal portions of lavender flowers, catmint, marjoram, bay leaves, and chamomile, then strain it. Mix with the powder and use like nose drops.
Note: Has a very cleansing effect, clears out the paranasal sinuses and the frontal sinus and brings back the sense of smell that has been lost (through the illness).

❀ Powdered black cumin seeds or even oil rubbed into the nose should help against headaches, as well as cataract in the beginning stage.

TWO RECIPES AGAINST EARACHES

❀ Drip a few drops of black cumin oil with a pipette directly into the auditory canal and massage a bit of oil into the skin behind the ear.

❀ Put 2 tablespoons of finely ground black cumin seeds into 2 tablespoons of black cumin oil that has been slightly warmed and fry them in it. Strain and let cool off. Spread this oil extract into the ear 3 x a day. This should also have an effect on the sinuses.

OLD TIME-TESTED RECIPES FOR FEVER

❀ For "recurrent fever," take 2 parts black cumin seeds and 1 part parsley seeds in warmed wine "to sweat and drive away the fever."

❀ Finely crush black cumin seeds, mix with mercury juice, and form into little "pills," of which 2 – 3 should be taken every day.

Furthermore, for the treatment of acute symptoms and to increase the body's resistance, drink the tea mixture made of black cumin, liquorice, and anise, sweetened with honey, apportioned throughout the day. Warm milk with black cumin oil and honey is particularly recommended for children: 1 teaspoon each of oil and honey in 1 cup of milk. The black cumin syrup with honey, garlic, and ginger is also an expectorant and has a very cleansing effect in general.

Further Applications in the Head Area

Toothaches and inflammations of the gums

The accompanying curative effect of black cumin for complaints and diseases in the mouth area can be explained on the basis of its anti-bacterial, anti-inflammatory, and pain-killing qualities. Old recipes have been handed down from various cultures, and these have been supplemented by new experiences. Here is a selection from them:

- ❀ The simplest: rub the painful spot with 1 – 2 drops of black cumin oil
- ❀ Use black cumin oil (in place of the usual sunflower oil) for rinsing the mouth with oil: take 1 teaspoon of black cumin oil in the morning, thoroughly "suck" it through the teeth, and "chew it." Afterwards, the oil must be spit out and the mouth thoroughly cleaned since the oil has taken on many toxins from the oral cavity.
- ❀ Stir crushed black cumin seeds into a paste with olive oil and rub the teeth and gums with it.
- ❀ Apple-cider vinegar can also be used in place of the olive oil.
- ❀ Warm 1 cup of apple-cider vinegar and let 2 tablespoons of finely ground black cumin seeds cook in it for another 5 minutes. Strain the mixture. Use for several days to extensively rinse out the mouth.
- ❀ Pulverize 1 teaspoon each of black cumin seeds, anise seeds, and cloves into a fine powder and mix together. After brushing the teeth, put 1 teaspoon of this mixture into the mouth without adding any liquid to it. Soak it well with saliva and "bath" the gums in it until the mixture can be swallowed.
- ❀ According to an old Oriental recipe, this spice powder should also help against headaches that radiate from the eyes.

Painful eyes

Because of an overstraining of the eyes, above all as a result of work at the computer monitor, painful eyes have become a widespread phenomenon of our times that can frequently also contribute to headaches. Here are some remedies:

❀ Eye compresses with black cumin: boil 1 tablespoon of black cumin seeds in 1 cup of water. Let draw for 10 minutes and then strain.

❀ As a supportive measure, the temples can be rubbed with black cumin oil before going to sleep.

❀ In Ayurvedic medicine, a decoction of *kalonji* (black onion seed alias black cumin), *curcuma* (tumeric), and *kassumar* ginger is recommended against clouded vision on the basis of inflamed mucous membranes (to which we would give the modern term of "conjunctivitis").

Headaches

The use of black cumin against headaches was already mentioned in an entire series of old healing books and substantiated by a great variety of recipes. For modern research, the effect takes place on several levels such as:

• through the regulation of the hormonal system
• through vasodilation (effect of the prostaglandins)
• through increased elimination of uric acid.

In acute cases, 1 teaspoon of black cumin oil can be taken twice or a total of 6 capsules daily, but for not more than 3 weeks. This therapy can be effectively supported by giving up as much as possible.

❀ In addition, the temples can be rubbed with black cumin oil. This promotes detoxification and better circulation through the essential active ingredients.

TIME-TESTED EUROPEAN RECIPES

* ❀ Mix pulverized black cumin seeds with rose vinegar or apple-cider vinegar into a paste and apply to the forehead and temples.
* ❀ In place of rose vinegar, rose honey can also be used.
* ❀ The effect is said to be even stronger when "blue-lily oil" (iris versicolor) is added.
* ❀ For headaches caused by the cold, rubbing the pulverized seeds or the oil into the nose is helpful.

ORIENTAL SPICE POWDER

* ❀ Mix 50 grams each of ground black cumin seeds
* ❀ ground anise seeds
* ❀ clove powder

with each other and store in a jar in a cool place. Take 1 teaspoon without liquids twice daily, before breakfast and lunch; soak it with saliva in the mouth until it can be swallowed.

* ❀ Also helps against toothaches and inflammation of the gums.

A 45-year-old woman had suffered for about 15 years from chronic migraine headaches, which at times had caused her to have an intensive dazed feeling. After a daily ingestion of 4 – 6 black cumin oil capsules, a distinct improvement of the complaints occurred after just 3 weeks.

Weak Concentration

Concentration disorders that initially manifest themselves as relatively harmless but bothersome forgetfulness, yet may also lead to a state of confusion and actual senile dementia at an older age, can be helped with an increased supply of essential fatty acids and the resulting stimulation of prostaglandin E1's activity. This has a regulating effect on the brain functions, the nerve conduction, and the release of transmitter and messenger substances. The result of this is a far-reaching influence on behavior. Black cumin has an additional effect because of its essential substances. For this reason, it is recommended that black cumin oil be taken in a daily dose of 3 capsules on a regular and timely, meaning *preventive*, basis.

❀ As support for weak concentration, 1 teaspoon of the spice-powder mixture of black cumin seeds, anise, and cloves can be taken 2 x a day (see recipe under *Headaches*).
❀ For weak concentration, mental exhaustion, and confusion, the essential black cumin oil (5 drops, possibly mixed with essential lavender oil and a citrus scent) in a fragrance lamp or for inhalation has proved to have a very good effect but should not be used on a continual basis.

Hyperactivity in children

Concentration disorders in children are often connected with the so-called "fidgeter syndrome." This is physically expressed by extreme mobility, uncoordinated movements, and fidgeting. In the psychological area, not only a lack of concentration is expressed but also extreme nervousness and sometimes even conspicuous, aggressive behavior.

Mr. Wilhelm H., 81 years old, suffered from decompensated cardiac insufficiency, extreme weakness, and confusion. Within one week's time, his condition had dramatically worsened: he was confused and fell down each time he tried to get out of bed. Since he has was in need of care to an extensive degree and could no longer remain in his apartment, his relatives had him move in with them.

As an initial dose, he was given 1 teaspoon of black cumin oil daily. After 3 weeks, the dosage was switched to 3 x 1 capsule a day. After about 10 days, the confusion began to improved. It completely disappeared after one month's time. The extreme physical weakness had already improved to such an extent after one week that Mr. H. no longer fell down. After 1 month, he sometimes even felt himself capable of climbing a flight of stairs.

After 2 months, he stopped taking the black cumin oil. Just 14 days later, the first symptoms of confusion appeared again. After 3 days, during which Mr. H. received 1 teaspoon of black cumin oil 3 x daily, his condition improved again. Now he takes 1 black cumin oil capsule 3 x a day and—considering the circumstances—he is doing well.

Through an increased supply of essential fatty acids and the regulating effect of prostaglandin E1 on the brain and nerves, it has been possible to achieve tangible progress. Not only is concentration supported but the general physical and mental functional capacity is increased.

Dosage for schoolchildren:
- ❀ In the first 3 weeks, 1/2 teaspoon of black cumin oil 2 x a day or 2 x 1 capsule.
- ❀ Afterwards, 1 – 2 capsules a day as a maintenance dose under observation.

Disturbed Sleep

Sleep problems that are manifested as either difficulties in falling asleep or in sleeping through the night without waking up very frequently have psychological causes or are brought about by over-stimulation of the nerves. Ayurvedic medicine has known of the stimulating and simultaneously pain-relieving influence of black cumin on the nervous system and the senses. It makes use of black cumin for "*vata* disorders of the nervous system," which are expressed in restlessness and hyperactivity. In addition to the generally regulative effect of black cumin, its bitter principles serve as a specific nerve tonic.

Time-tested recipes

❀ *Strong nerve tea:*
Infuse 1 cup of black cumin seeds with 1 liter of hot water. Let draw for 10 minutes, then strain. Drink the liquid at intervals throughout the entire day: start in the morning on an empty stomach before breakfast, and drink the last cup 1 – 2 hours before going to sleep.

Who doesn't remember having
❀ *Hot milk with honey?*
Stir 1 teaspoon of black cumin oil and 1 teaspoon of honey into 1 cup of warm milk. Drink just before going to sleep.
❀ Rub the temples with black cumin oil and then turn off the light ...

Gynecological Complaints

In Ayurveda, in the Arabian countries, and in earlier times in Central Europe as well, the effect of black cumin on menstrual complaints and for fertility, birth (as an ecbolic for contractions), and lactation, and also for sepsis (puerperal fever) in India, has been handed down for a long time and confirmed by many recipes. More recent studies have been able to prove a regulation of the hormonal system through the tissue hormones. Also among the modern areas of application are the premenstrual syndrome and complaints of menopause.

Important note: *Black cumin should not be taken during pregnancy since the prostaglandins could possibly cause a dilation of the mouth of the womb and therefore possible premature labor.*

FOR MENSTRUAL DISORDERS

❀ Drink 1 cup of black cumin tea (1 teaspoon of black cumin seed per cup) 2 x daily

❀ For relaxation of the abdominal musculature and the uterus: dissolve 1/2 teaspoon of the fatty oil or 5 – 8 drops of essential black cumin oil in 1 liter of hot water and use to make warm abdominal compresses

❀ Old Arabian recipe: mix finely ground black cumin, anise, and cloves in equal portions and take 1 teaspoon of the mixture *without liquids* before meals (soak in saliva until it can be swallowed).

FOR WOMEN IN CHILDBED WITH DEFICIENT LACTATION

❀ Drink 1 cup of black cumin tea 3 x daily

*FOR DISTURBED BODILY SECRETIONS AND LACK OF APPETITE
AFTER DELIVERY*

❀ Black cumin, caraway, anise, *ajowan* (a type of parsley seed), *Carum sativum* (type of caraway), *Anethum sowa* (type of dill), *Methi*, coriander, ginger, pods and roots of *Pippali* (long pepper), leadwort, *habusha* (an aromatic substance), dried pulp of *badri* (jujube berries), and *kamala* powder (lotus seeds) are cooked into a syrup together with molasses, milk, and *ghee* (clarified butter). Take 1 teaspoon of this mixture every morning (the original recipe states 1 drachma = 3.75 grams).

FOR COMPLAINTS OF MENOPAUSE

❀ Drink black cumin tea on a regular basis.
❀ Take the strong powder of black cumin, anise, and cloves on an empty stomach every morning.
❀ Take black cumin oil/capsules as a treatment for up to 3 months.

Metabolic Disturbances

Metabolic disturbances are understood here to be all deviations from the normal metabolic processes. In this respect, acute forms are often triggered by an improper diet while chronic diseases can be induced by a genetically based enzyme deficiency. The organs of the stomach and intestines, liver and gallbladder, pancreas (diabetes), kidneys, and bladder are are primarily afflicted. Metabolic disorders are also at least contributing factors to a variety of rheumatic illnesses, as well as vascular diseases (arteriosclerosis).

This is a "wide field" in which black cumin seeds can germinate! It has traditionally been known as a pleasant-tasting and easily digestible seasoning for bread and other foods, primarily in the Orient but also in Europe for a good many years and is still in use today. Black cumin also appears to be an extremely popular remedy for vague "stomach-aches." Its digestant and flatulence-inhibiting action, but also proven effect against more serious complaints in the digestive tract, has been explained in the meantime mainly because of the saponin melanthin and the bitter principle nigellin. Both components are known for their strong eliminatory quality, which serves both intestinal cleansing as well as an increased secretion of urine (because they break down excessive acids within the body). Bitter principles also have a stimulating effect on the liver and gallbladder (fatty metabolism) and an anti-spasmodic effect on chronic inflammations and the formation of stones (gallbladder, kidneys, and bladder).

In addition, the essential components in black cumin, nigellone and thymoquinone, have a generally relaxing and pain-relieving effect. Thymoquinone is also a choleretic (stimulates the gallbladder).

Gastrointestinal Complaints

Among these are all types of digestive complaints, diffuse stomach-aches, flatulence, heartburn, a sensation of fullness, diarrhea (also when it is accompanied by vomiting), and constipation. A short-term treatment with black cumin in the form of specific recipes is required for acute symptoms of this type. For complaints that tend to be chronic or frequently recurring, a treatment with black cumin oil or capsules for several weeks is recommended. To fight against intestinal fungi, a detoxification treatment as a measure to accompany therapy for symbiotic management is advisable.

TIME-TESTED TEA RECIPE FOR DIGESTIVE PROBLEMS

❀ The simplest recipe against flatulence, diffuse stomach pains, and constipation: Infuse 1 gram (about 1 teaspoon) of crushed black cumin seeds with 1/4 liter of water that is no longer boiling hot. Let draw for 10 minutes and then strain. Drink 1 cup 2 – 3 times a day, at best unsweetened, between meals. Also affects an increased elimination and is beneficial for gallbladder problems.
Tea-herbal mixtures
❀ *Arabian recipe*: Infuse equal parts of black cumin seeds, fennel, and peppermint with hot water. Let draw for 10 minutes and then strain. Drink 1 cup between meals 2 – 3 times a day.
❀ *European variation*: Use equal parts of *angelica root* and *cinquefoil* in addition to the black cumin seeds.
❀ *New variation*: Drip 3 – 7 drops of black cumin oil into each cup of herbal tea from the two recipes above.
❀ *New combination method*: Infuse equal parts of anise and fennel seeds with hot water. Let cool down to about 30°C. Add 1 teaspoon of black cumin oil. Drink 3 – 4 cups a day between meals.

Suggestions for ALL-ROUND TREATMENT OF STOMACH PAINS
(when accompanied by a sensation of fullness and flatulence):

- ❀ *Externally*: apply abdominal pack or compresses that have been soaked in a mixture of warmed apple-cider vinegar and pulverized black cumin or a few drops of black cumin oil.
- ❀ *Internally*: Drink a tea mixture of black cumin, fennel, and peppermint several times a day and add 3 – 7 drops of black cumin oil to each cup.
- ❀ Tonic for more severe complaints: Boil 2 parts apple-cider vinegar with 1 part ground black cumin seeds and add 1 part black cumin oil at the end. Take 1 teaspoon 2 x daily before meals. Also helps against intestinal parasites.

For colic and diarrhea with vomiting
(also for possible food poisoning)

- ❀ Infuse equal parts of black cumin seeds and cloves with hot water. Drink 1 cup of this 3 x daily without sweetener.
- ❀ For longer-lasting complaints, additionally take 1/2 teaspoon or 1 capsule of black cumin oil several times a day.
- ❀ In the Ayurvedic medicine, black cumin seeds are roasted and taken in a mixture with molasses against vomiting.

Recipe with warm milk and honey
(suited above all for children to sweeten the stomach-ache)

The Ayurvedic, Arabian, and European tradition is familiar with and recommends taking black cumin oil in lukewarm milk for all types of digestive complaints. The milk has an additional calming effect on the afflicted gastric mucous membrane.

- ❀ Universal recipe, above all for children: Warm 1 cup of milk, sweeten with 1 teaspoon of honey, and stir in 1/2 teaspoon of black cumin oil. Divide to take at 3 meals and drink slowly.
- ❀ Also helps against stomach cramps and heartburn.

*AUSTRIAN FOLK RECIPE FOR A TINCTURE AGAINST DIGESTIVE
COMPLAINTS* (suited for adults and not children):
Pour 1/2 liter of good fruit schnapps in a wide-necked bottle together with 150 grams of crushed black cumin seeds
and place next to a window for 14 days. Strain and dilute with
distilled water to an alcohol content of about 36%. Take 1
tablespoon as required.

AYURVEDIC BLACK CUMIN RECIPES

❀ *Against lack of appetite and weight loss*
   Mix black cumin seeds, caraway, black pepper, raisins,
   tamarind pulp, pomegranate juice, and *sanchal* salt with
   molasses and honey into a very powerful and pleasant-
   tasting syrup. Take 1 teaspoon before meals (the original recipe states that 1 drachma = 3.75 grams).
❀ *For a sensation of fullness and to promote weight loss*
   Mix 2 parts of black cumin seed and 2 parts *ajowan* (a
   type of cumin) with 1 part *lakh mugsul* and crush into a
   powder. Take about 2 grams (1/2 drachma) a day.
❀ *Jawarish-ai-kammon*
   (For diarrhea, dyspepsia, and sour belching)
   Black cumin, white and black pepper, cinnamon bark,
   leaves of the ruewort (Ruta graveoleus), ginger conserve
   and myrobalans conserve are boiled into confection with
   sugar and rose syrup. Take 1 teaspoon of this 3 x a day.
   Also helps against bad breath.

GENERAL INGESTION RECOMMENDATIONS

The overall symptoms of disorders in the gastro-intestinal
tract with a tendency towards chronic complaints can be
treated by taking black cumin oil or capsules according to
the usual dosage suggestions:

❀ Initial dose for 3 weeks
   1 teaspoon of oil solution 3 x daily (1/2 teaspoon 2 x daily
   for children) for 3 weeks

❀ As a continuation or preventive dose 3 – 4 capsules a day (1 – 2 for children).

The following case history of one of Dr. Refai's patients illustrates the effectiveness of this treatment.

> *A 65-year-old woman suffered from a variety of complaints such as chronic stomach-ache and digestive disorders, underweight, and a general lack of vitality. As a treatment, she took 2 – 3 teaspoons of black cumin oil every day and also rubbed her stomach with the oil. Already after 3 weeks, it was possible to determine an obvious relief of her digestive disorders and an improvement of her general condition.*

Parasites, fungi, & co. in the intestines

Numerous European folk recipes from the 17th and 18th centuries have been handed down against "belly-ache and abdominal worms":
❀ Take 1 tablespoon of ground black cumin seeds with 1 cup of warm water in the morning on an empty stomach for several days.
❀ Drink crushed black cumin seeds in warmed wine for a number of days (can also be boiled in wine beforehand). Healing effect: "stills the ache and drives the worms out of the body."

As a remedy against intestinal parasites, the following can be used externally:
❀ Boil in vinegar and then spread on the navel.
❀ Or pulverize and mix with wormwood juice to make a plaster for the lower abdomen.

Warm 1 cup of apple-cider vinegar with 1/2 cup of finely ground black cumin seeds. Add 1/2 cup black cumin oil to this and boil on a low flame until it takes on a syrupy consistency. Store in a cool place. Take 1 tablespoon of this mixture before the meals. Helps against intestinal fungi, as well as against chronic intestinal inflammation and flatulence.

For intestinal fungi, a fundamental detoxification treatment according to the guidelines as described in detail in the chapter "Prevention Is Better Than Healing" is recommended.

❀ Take 3 teaspoons of black cumin oil or 6 capsules a day for 3 weeks.

❀ Afterwards, reduce to 3 capsules.

Liver and Gallbladder Complaints

Black cumin, through its bitter principles and saponins for strengthening the liver function and promoting bile secretion, effectively supplements the important role of the essential fatty acids for the entire fatty metabolism.

OLD ARABIAN RECIPE FOR A BITTER TINCTURE
(serves to strengthen the liver and stomach)

Mix together:
* 1 tablespoon of ground black cumin seeds
* 1 tablespoon of bitter liver tincture (use dandelion or, as an alternative, 1/2 teaspoon of Syrian oregano or a comparable, slightly peppery sort)
* 1 teaspoon of honey

and take 1 teaspoon of this mixture every morning over a longer period of time (about 2 months).

TEA FOR PREVENTION OF GALLSTONES

* For the simplest recipe, crush 1 teaspoon of black cumin seeds and pour 1/4 liter of hot water over them. Let draw for 15 minutes and then strain. Drink 2 cups of this every day.
* This is effectively supported by mixing it with celandine.

Increased cholesterol level

Cholesterol as a precursor to bile acid fulfills an important function in the fatty metabolism and, if the values are increased, can lead to changes in the vessels and coronary heart disease. It has been proved that a high portion of polyunsaturated fatty acids in the food (black cumin oil!) can lower the level of cholesterol in the blood. *Beta-sitosterol*, which has also been found in black cumin and has a vegetable source, is said to have a distinct cholesterol-lowering effect as well.

The effect of black cumin is additionally supported by taking antioxidants.

Ingestion recommendation: Take 2 – 3 black cumin oil capsules with vitamin E, which also strengthens the heart and circulation, every day for several weeks.

Diabetes

The effect of black cumin on type II diabetes (diabetes of old age) can be explained through the sinking of the blood-sugar level and—because it strengthens the immune system—the control of allergic factors. Black cumin can also be used as an accompanying treatment, whereby it only is effective when taken over a longer period of time.

❀ Take 1/2 – 1 teaspoons or 1 – 2 capsules 3 x a day.

❀ *Important note:* Since the danger of a blood-sugar level that is too low may arise, it is absolutely necessary that a doctor checks the blood-sugar levels on a regular basis!

OLD ARABIAN RECIPE AGAINST EXCESSIVELY HIGH BLOOD SUGAR

Finely grind equal portions of:

❀ black cumin seeds
true elecampane root
Syrian oregano
pomegranate peels

and mix with each other. Store the powder in a cool place. Take 1 tablespoon of it 15 minutes before each meal.

Kidney and Bladder Diseases

Because of the detoxifying and eliminatory, anti-spasmodic and anti-inflammatory qualities of black cumin, excellent healing effects can take place. This is also reflected in the many special recipes.

Moreover, black cumin is considered to be a good pepper substitute for people suffering from kidney disease.

TEA FOR STIMULATING THE KIDNEYS AND BLADDER
(increased urination)

* Infuse 1 teaspoon of crushed black cumin seeds with 1/4 liter of water that has stopped boiling. Let draw for 15 minutes and strain. Drink 2 cups of this a day. Especially well-suited for preventing renal gravel.
* Effectively supported by mixing with golden rod and horsetail.

OLD "DIURETIC" RECIPES

* Take 1 tablespoon of crushed black cumin seeds in the morning on an empty stomach
* For several days in a row, drink black cumin seeds that have been crushed and boiled in wine.

RECIPES AGAINST DIFFICULTIES IN URINATING (according to Tabernaemontanus' Herbal Book, 18th century)

Crush 2 ounces of black cumin seeds, mix with 3 ounces of sugar, and pour a good, old white wine over it; fill into a screw-cap bottle and let stand. Later, let simmer for 4 hours, cool, and strain. Drink 4 ounces of this mixture warm in the morning on an empty stomach and in the evening 2 hours before going to bed.

ARABIAN RECIPE AGAINST KIDNEY STONES (PREVENTION)

Mix together:

❀ 1 tablespoon crushed black cumin seeds
   1 tablespoon honey
   1 teaspoon crushed garlic cloves or ginger.

Take 1 teaspoon of this mixture before each meal. Store in a screw-lid jar in the refrigerator (keeps for 15 days).

FURTHER INGESTION RECOMMENDATIONS IN THE CASE OF RENAL-GRAVEL FORMATION

❀ For less severe complaints, take 1 tablespoon of black cumin seeds before breakfast.

❀ Take 1 teaspoon of black cumin oil 2 – 3 x daily or 3 x 2 capsules.

❀ Prepare mate tea, let cool down to 30°C, add 3 – 5 drops of black cumin oil. Drink several cups a day.

❀ Rub the area of the kidneys with black cumin oil.

❀ Even better, if you have the time, are *kidney wraps*:
heat 2 tablespoons of olive oil, stir in 2 tablespoons of finely ground black cumin seeds, and let draw for 15 minutes. Put mixture on a cotton cloth and apply for about 20 minutes (wrap a large towel around you for protection).

BLADDER INFLAMMATION

This infection is frequently triggered by germs from the intestines that have reached the bladder through the ureter so that a longer-term *intestinal detoxification* over a period of 3 – 6 months can eliminate this problem in many cases.

❀ As a supportive measure, massage the lower abdomen with black cumin oil and drink plenty of liquids such as black cumin tea sweetened with honey.

Hemorrhoids

Hemorrhoids are actually a vascular disease that allows varicose veins to occur on the anus because of vein dilation. Since poor eating habits, constipation, and intestinal toxins are contributing factors to this disorder, just taking black cumin oil can have a very good effect on it.

Here are further traditional recipes for internal and external treatment:

❀ Mash black cumin seeds with cane sugar in a ratio of 1:1 and take a tablespoons of it at a time. *Drink plenty of liquids afterwards!*

❀ Clean the inflamed and itching spots and rub with black cumin oil.

❀ Take a hip bath (15 ml of black cumin oil to 1 liter of water).

❀ Make black cumin ash according to an old recipe by letting black cumin seeds smolder to ash in an iron pan (without fat) and apply this to the cleaned hemorrhoids.

Two Arabian recipes for vein creams

❀ Let black cumin seed smolder into ash according to the recipe above and mix into a cream with 1 tablespoon of black cumin oil. Spread onto the hemorrhoids on a regular basis.

Suitable for varicose ulcers:

❀ Let black cumin seed smolder in an iron pain and mix into a paste with 2 tablespoons of henna fat. Apply to the well-cleaned leg and wrap with a sterile bandage after it has dried. Renew 1 – 2 x daily.

Rheumatic Disorders and Arthritic Pain

Rheumatism is a generalized disorder with a multitude of causes that have not yet been completely clarified, among which are metabolic disturbances and allergic factors. The essential fatty acids contained in black cumin oil, as well as its immunoregulatory and anti-inflammatory substances, contribute at least to relief of the pain. This is also valid for its external applications.

OLD ARABIC RECIPE FOR ARTHRITIC PAIN

Carefully heat 2 tablespoons of black cumin oil, add 2 tablespoons of freshly ground black cumin seeds, and stir until the mixture has a creamy consistency. This paste should be applied:
* cooled for *inflammatory* processes
* slightly *heated* for *degenerative* processes.

RECOMMENDATIONS FOR APPLICATION

* Internally: the standard dosage of 2 teaspoons of oil solution or 6 capsules daily for 3 weeks.
* Externally: Place a warm, dry cloth on the painful area for 10 minutes and then rub in the slightly heated black cumin oil.
* Avoid extreme cold and heat.

A 50-year-old woman had suffered from a rheumatic disorder that had become chronic for about 10 years. She had intense pains in all the joints, particularly in the hips, knees, elbows, and wrists. She was in such a poor condition that she could only get up and walk with someone else's help.

After she had taken 3 teaspoons of black cumin oil every day for 4 weeks and had rubbed oil on the afflicted areas on a regular basis at the same time, a definite reduction of the pain occurred and the patient could slowly get up again and walk on her own.

Bruises and Injuries

Black cumin oil has a local effect on the skin when applied externally and, because its components can penetrate into the tissue, on the deeper-lying layers as well. Through the effect of the essential substances, there is initially a detoxification and better circulation within the tissue. Then the anti-inflammatory influence of prostaglandin E1 begins. In addition, black cumin oil has the ability of more quickly eliminating skin cells that have died and accelerating healing processes. For this reason, black cumin oil can also be used for bruises, contusions, sprains, and similar injuries, and even for minor burns.

RECOMMENDATIONS FOR USE:

* For affected skin areas, rub on some black cumin oil, either undiluted or mixed with tea tree oil several times a day. *Don't heat* oil for this application.
* St. John's Wort oil and wheat germ oil are very well-suited as carrier oils.
* For minor burns, black cumin oil can be mixed with St. John's Wort oil and some essential lavender oil and applied to the wound—apply black cumin oil undiluted in case of sunburn.
* Put 5 – 7 drops of essential oil in 1 liter of water and place compresses that have been soaked in it on the wound several times a day, if possible.
* Use with warm water for muscle cramps.

BEAUTIFUL
SKIN & HAIR

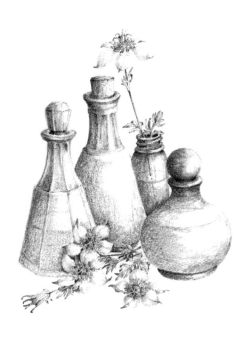

Black Cumin in Cosmetics, Body Care, and Hygiene

The Skin

Black cumin also has a long tradition in the area of beauty care—to what other secret could the ancient Egyptians have most likely owed their famous, even "bronze complexion"? In the Orient and at latest since the 1st century in Europe, as recorded by Pliny, there are many recipes for maintaining and obviously also for restoring beauty with the help of black cumin. The seeds are also suitable for cleansing the skin: they are mixed with water or apple-cider vinegar and applied to the skin for deep cleansing; healing earth can also be used along with it for compresses and facial masks. The concentrated black cumin oil naturally possesses the greatest degree of effectiveness. In the 18th century, Tabernaemontanus mentioned a recipe with *Melanthium oleum*, which is made with sesame oil. This helps against skin impurities and makes the facial skin smoother.

Not only problem skin, but also healthy skin is dependent on an adequate supply of healthy and nutritive natural substances to a large extent. Vegetable oils with a high portion of polyunsaturated fatty acids internally provide for:
- detoxification of the organism
- regeneration of the intestines
- regulation of the hormonal system
- harmonization of the immune system

and all of these processes are obviously reflected in the condition of the skin as well. In addition, these oils have a local effect since they penetrate deep into the skin tissue and simultaneously have a relaxing and vitalizing effect, which is very beneficial for skin that is intensely stressed and tired. In addition, there is also a detoxifying and anti-inflammatory effect for skin impurities. Because of their high portion of essential fatty acids, black cumin oil, evening primrose oil, and borage oil—and, according to the most recent research, also hempseed oil, oil from rose-hips, and the seeds of the black currant—are all excellent cosmetics. When *natural* vitamin E (tocopherol) is added as an antioxidant, the process of cell aging is slowed down, which also becomes evident in the appearance of the skin: cell renewal is supported, the connective tissue remains strong, and the skin becomes smooth and elastic.

FIRST THE CLEANSING ...

* Nigella bran for impure skin: mix black cumin seeds that have been roughly ground or crushed with a mortar and then "rub down" the affected skin areas with it. Afterwards, thoroughly rinse with lukewarm water.
* For skin that tends to be dry, the black cumin seeds can also be mixed with some black cumin oil instead of water.
* Facial steambaths with black cumin (seeds, fatty oil, and essential oil) have a supportive effect that also beneficially influences the respiratory tract and the eyes.

ARABIAN RECIPE AGAINST ACNE AND OTHER SKIN PROBLEMS

* Mix 1 cup of freshly ground black cumin seeds and 1/2 cup of ground pomegranate peels with each other, pour in 1/2 cup of apple-cider vinegar, and heat on a low flame to 50°C. Stir well and then add 1 tablespoon of black cumin oil. Apply to the affected parts of the skin. This mixture will keep for 3 weeks when stored in a cool place.
* Mix freshly ground black cumin seeds and finely ground wheat or wheat germ in a 1:1 ration. Add sesame oil and stir to make a paste. Apply in the evening so that it can have its effect on the skin overnight.
* Helpful against itching during the healing of inflamed areas of the skin is a mixture of 100 ml jojoba oil to which 20 drops each of black cumin oil and tea tree oil have been added. The tea tree oil must be of a very good quality, if possible from a wild-growing source or from control-

led organic cultivation so that skin irritations do not occur because of an excessive cineole content.

BEAUTY RECIPES FROM *1001 NIGHTS*

❀ Mix black cumin oil in equal parts with almond oil and olive oil. Apply directly to the skin after it has been cleansed. People used to then sit out in the sun for an hour with this mixture on their faces and wipe it off afterwards. The skin gratefully responds with a very youthful and smooth appearance.

❀ *Modern version:* Use a mixture of black cumin oil with almond oil and jojoba oil, which is actually a wax with very good skin-care qualities—and you probably shouldn't sit out in the sun!

❀ *Facial mask:* Mix 1 tablespoon of black cumin oil with 1 tablespoon of honey. Apply this to the cleansed facial skin and let this take effect for 15 minutes. Rinse off with lukewarm water. Has a very relaxing effect, and the skin feels smooth once again.

BEAUTY RECIPES FOR EVERY DAY

At the moments there are relatively few ready-made cosmetic products offered with black cumin oil. However, you can easily prepare them on your own by enriching either your personal favorite cream or body lotion with a few drops of black cumin oil. Further suggestions for beauty care are found in the following recipes:

❀ Facial balm: Put 50 ml of black cumin oil and 50 ml of jojoba oil in a water-bath, together with 10 grams of beeswax, and warm to about 50°C until the wax liquifies. Mix the ingredients well and let cool. Jojoba oil is a liquid wax that hardly oxidates and does not become rancid as a result. This makes it an ideal carrier oil, also for hair care. According to personal preferences and/or skin type, a few drops of essential oil like bergamot, grapefruit, and cinnamon can be added for tonicizing or rose, sandalwood, and chamomile for sensitive skin.

FACIAL OILS

- ❊ Using the basis of black cumin oil and jojoba oil, you can also prepare a facial oil instead of a cream. In this case, it is recommended that you add essential oils such as 10 drops of tea tree oil and 10 drops of lavender oil or chamomile oil to 100 ml of fatty vegetable oil.
- ❊ You can mix 15 – 20 drops of *essential* black cumin oil with 100 ml of a lotion or a vegetable oil that you tolerate well.

BODY OILS AND MASSAGE OILS

- ❊ You can also easily prepare body oils, which can be used after the bath or for massage purposes, according to the directions above. Black cumin oil strengthens the connective tissue, stimulates the blood supply to the skin, and has a tonicizing and smoothing effect on the skin.
- ❊ By adding selected essential oils, you can influence whether the massage should have more of a stimulating effect (for example, with citrus scents, rosemary) or whether it has a more relaxing effect (for example, with lavender, geranium, clary sage).
- ❊ All oils keep for a considerably longer time when 1 tablespoon of wheat germ oil is added as an antioxidant.

ADDITIONAL RECOMMENDATIONS

- ❊ For the general revitalization of exhausted and dull, pale skin, add 5 ml of black cumin oil to the bath water several times a week.
- ❊ During times of intensive stress, the external application can be effectively supported by a preventive treatment of taking 1/2 teaspoon of black cumin oil or 3 capsules per day.

Hair Care

Just like the skin, the hair also reflects the general condition of the body. Taking black cumin oil internally should therefore also contribute to healthy hair by regulating various bodily functions. However, there are also a few outstanding old recipes for its external application.

Arabian Recipe for Strong Hair Growth

✿ Grind 1 handful of black cumin seeds and mix into a paste with some warmed olive oil. Apply to the scalp and hair until the substance has dried (takes 1/2 – 1 hour). Wash out thoroughly.

✿ Mix equal parts of black cumin oil with onion seed oil and olive oil and heat a bit. Rub into scalp and hair, let it take effect for at least 1/2 hour, and then wash out thoroughly.

From Culpeper's Complete Herbal (17th century)

✿ Infuse 1 handful of black cumin seeds crushed with the mortar with 1 quarter liter of olive oil. Pour into a firmly closing jar and put in a warm place for 2 weeks. Strain through gauze cloth and squeeze the seeds well. Keep in a dark bottle. Massage into the hair each time before washing, let it have an effect on the scalp, and then wash out thoroughly.

✿ In place of the olive oil, burdock root oil, apricot oil, or hazelnut oil can be put to good use.

Secret Recipe against Hair Loss

✿ Wash the hair every second day, dry with a towel or let it dry in the air. Massage black cumin oil into the hair. Let it take effect for 1/2 hour, then thoroughly wash out hair.

✿ Take 2 teaspoons of black cumin oil daily as support from within.

Black Cumin for Hygiene

According to old tradition, black cumin seeds used to be filled into little linen sacks and placed in the linen cupboard or in beds. This kept away the cockroaches, fleas, lice, and other bugs. There is a traditional custom in all of India in which crushed *kalonji* seeds are sprinkled between fabrics and scarves. Black cumin seeds were also burned so that their smoke kept away not only insects but also snakes and scorpions; the custom of treating scorpion stings with black cumin has also been handed down in India. As we have already heard, in the Orient black cumin has had the reputation of banishing the "evil eye," while Europeans were satisfied with keeping away witches with it.

A paste made of 4 parts finely ground black cumin seeds and 1 part apple-cider vinegar can be applied to the skin and hair against head lice and skin parasites (like itch mites). Let it dry and take effect for several hours, if possible, before washing it out.

For an additional disinfecting and anti-inflammatory effect, rub the skin with black cumin oil that has had a few drops of essential tea tree oil and lavender oil or chamomile oil added to it. This helps against insect bites or even serves as an insect repellent when it is applied in due time.

More for the sake of completeness, the use of black cumin seeds and oil in veterinary medicine should be mentioned here as well; the grist that occurs during production is also mixed into feed. This use of black cumin has primarily been handed down from the Near East, yet it was also familiar in Central Europe several centuries ago. Among the areas of application are stable dust allergy and nettle rash in horses, weed in cows, and pigeon pox, as well as an increased fertility and weight in feeder poultry.

Perhaps more interesting for the reader is its use for dogs and cats against fleas and other parasites. A mixture of black cumin oil and tea tree oil can be spread on the animal's fur in order to keep away undesired guests. Should a tick have settled on the skin, drip a bit of black cumin oil on it and carefully twist it out with tweezers. A few drops for the follow-up treatment prevent inflammation and accelerate the healing process.

BLACK CUMIN
IN THE KITCHEN

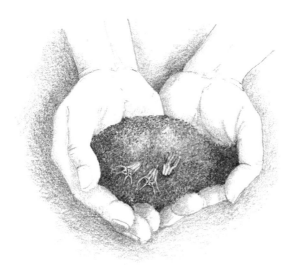

From Brotwurz to Kalonji

This versatile spice has at least as many names, which have been given to black cumin by the various cultures, as it has uses in the kitchen. As usual, they are not only imaginative but also quite confusing.

Despite the partly similar uses, there is no botanic relationship between *Nigella sativa* and *Carum carvi*, our customary spice caraway. This is why black cumin was given the name of "black coriander" in Germany, which points out its use there as a bread seasoning; however, it was also called "Roman cumin," which can be seen as a concession to its southern origins. Since the Middle Ages, the traditional German term among the common people has been *Brotwurz* or "bread-seasoning" in English

In English, black cumin has also been called "small fennel," which can probably be explained by its similarity to the finely pinnated leaves. Although the French call it *cumin noir* or *cumin faux* (meaning black or false cumin), they manage to get out of the problem quite elegantly by labelling it *toute épice*, the "universal spice."

Because of its digestant and flatulence-inhibiting effect, as well as, of course, for reasons of taste, black cumin has traditionally been used as a spice for baking bread in the Orient. It is put to use in many dishes there, and can be found in every kitchen. Although it is often coarsely ground or finely ground as an ingredient for bread, an even more popular way to use it is to sprinkle the whole seeds on flat breads or baked goods in the same way that poppy or sesame seeds are used. Because of its anti-bacterial qualities, it also serves to preserve food. Similar to how mustard or pepper seeds are used for spice pickles in Europe, a teaspoon of black cumin in the preserving jar can extend the shelf life of marinated vegetables. A further benefit of this method is the unusually spicy aroma. Sweet-and-sour pickles and chutney can also be given more pep with it—at any rate, black cumin is an outstanding substitute for pepper.

The Turkish name *çörekotu*, which can be translated into something like "grass for little pastry," indicates the old tradition as a bread seasoning, particularly its use in *börek*, a puff pastry filled with ewe's milk cheese. The Turkish stores in other countries also frequently offer flat breads sprinkled with *cörekotu*, and bakers of organic goods have likewise discovered the black cumin to be an interesting ingredient in breads made of grain like *kamut*, the old Egyptian wheat. There are German organic farmers who have recently begun to spice their meats and sausages—as well as vegetarian spelt spreads—with black cumin.

In the Indian kitchen, nigella seed is a very popular and frequently used spice. Here it is called *kalonji*—since its appearance is similar to that of onion seeds, it is sometimes offered as "black Indian onion seed." Very frequently it is confused with the two types of cumin, with the common *Cuminum cyminun* and quite understandably even more frequently with the *Cuminum nigrum*, the black cumin that is called *kala-jira* in India. In this manner, nigella-kalonji has received (certainly not undeserved) divine names like *Kalijeeri* or *Krishna-jiraka*! According to Ayurvedic teaching, the *kalonji* has the basic quality (*guna*) of "light and dry" and corresponds to the taste (*rasa*) of "hot and bitter." It is available in many Indian curry and spice mixtures such as in the five-seed *masala* together with cumin, fennel, black mustard seed, and fenugreek, giving the mixture the name of *panch phoron*—"five seeds."

As a spice, nigella seed can be well-employed in place of pepper. Although its taste is somewhat more bitter, it has more aroma and is not as hot as the latter; this also makes it the healthy alternative for people with sensitive gastric mucous membranes and kidney problems. The entire seed can be crushed with a mortar or put into a pepper mill. If a finer powder is preferred, a coffee mill is best suited for grinding the seeds. To intensify the aroma, the seeds first can be roasted in an iron pan without any fat in it before they are added to a dish. Black cumin is extremely versatile and can be added as a spice for soups, vegetable dishes and casseroles, sprinkled over salads, or mixed in with yoghurt and cottage cheese. Its taste fits in particularly well with *dal*, the Indian legume dish, but naturally with all the other legume dishes as well, with curries and chutneys, and with all types of cabbage, which simultaneously supports better digestion. Not only can an exotic flair be easily conjured up for meals by using black cumin—it also tastes good and is easily digestible. In short: this is the perfect ingredient for culinary healthy cooking.

In addition, a small amount (at most 1 teaspoon) of black cumin oil can be mixed with olive oil, for example, to refine salad dressings. However, do not cook or fry it along with hot dishes but drip it onto the food right at the end.

Some recipe suggestions will now follow below. However, they are mainly meant to stimulate new ideas. With black cumin, the spice with more than one-hundred components, an endless abundance of names, and the magic of 1001 Nights, there are no limits to your imagination—go ahead and try it out!

Cooking Recipes

CABBAGE À LA NIGELLE

Ingredients: 1 small cabbage
Cold-pressed sesame oil or thistle oil
Yeast seasoning
Black cumin seeds

Cut a small cabbage into fine strips and steam with an appropriate frying oil. Season according to taste, add some liquid, and let simmer on a small flame. Roast 1 tablespoon of black cumin seeds in an iron pan without fat, spread over the cabbage, which should not be cooked too soft, mix, and serve immediately.

INDIAN MUNGOBEAN YUSHA (SOUP)

Ingredients: 1 cup mungo beans (moong dal)
8 cups water
1/4 teaspoon curcuma powder
1 teaspoon stone salt powder
1 tablespoon sunflower or sunflower oil
1 teaspoon ground kalonji seeds
1/2 teaspoon ground kala-jira seeds
1 teaspoon freshly grated ginger
1 teaspoon finely chopped coriander leaves

Place the beans, which should been soaked in advance, into a large pot with the water and the curcuma powder. Cook on a small flame for about 30 minutes. Then add the salt. Crush the seeds in a mortar or grind into powder and fry together with the ginger in the oil. Put everything into the soup and let cook for a further 15 minutes. At the end, spread the finely chopped coriander leaves over it and let the soup draw a bit before serving.

Raw Food Recipes

ORIENTAL CUCUMBER SALAD WITH YOGHURT DRESSING

Ingredients: 1 salad cucumber
1 crushed clove of garlic
250 g thick (for example, Greek) yoghurt
1/2 teaspoon ground black cumin seeds
1 teaspoon finely chopped fresh mint
Salt

Finely grate and salt the salad cucumber. Mix the yoghurt with the black cumin and the mint, add the cucumber, and mix thoroughly. Serve immediately so that the dressing does not get watered down by the cucumber juice.

RAW SAUERKRAUT À LA RENATE

Ingredients: 150 g raw sauerkraut
1 teaspoon finely cut onion
1 tablespoon Styrian pumpkin seed oil
Freshly ground black cumin seeds
Salt

Chop the sauerkraut into smaller pieces and mix well with the other ingredients.

BLACK CUMIN SEED DRESSING

Ingredients: 1 – 1 1/2 teaspoons freshly ground black cumin
1 teaspoon sugar
1 pinch curcuma
5 tablespoons freshly squeezed lemon juice
120 ml walnut oil and olive oil

Mix the black cumin, sugar, curcuma, and lemon juice in a jar, close tightly, and shake well so that the sugar dissolves. Then add the walnut oil and olive oil and shake until all ingredients have mixed completely with each other. The dressing will keep for up to 2 weeks when stored in a cool place. It is used in the Orient for salads, as well as legume dishes.

BLACK CUMIN OIL VINAIGRETTE

Ingredients: 1 tablespoon "Aceto Balsamico" Vinegar
1/2 teaspoon coarse-grain mustard
Herb salt
2 tablespoons cold-pressed olive oil
1 teaspoon black cumin oil

Mix the mustard and herb salt with the vinegar and then add the oil.

BAKING RECIPES

The traditional method is to use 4 ounces of crushed or ground black cumin seeds for 3 pounds of flour. The seeds can be worked into the dough or sprinkled onto the bread. You can also add 1 tablespoon of black cumin oil to the dough to intensify the taste.

BLACK CUMIN WHOLE-GRAIN BREAD

Ingredients: 1 lb. whole-wheat flour
1 1/2 ounce finely or coarsely ground rye flour
Approx. 6 cups water
1 ounce yeast
1/3 ounce sea salt
1 2/3 ounces coarsely ground black cumin seeds
If desired, a bit of black cumin oil

Knead flour, yeast, and water into a medium-firm dough. Let rise for 15 minutes. Then mix into the spices (and, if desired, a few drops of black cumin oil), form a bread loaf or fill the dough into a baking tin. Let it rise for another 15 – 20 minutes and then bake for about 50 minutes at 230°C.

Yeast Rolls with Black Cumin

Ingredients: 1 lb. whole-wheat flour
1 2/3 ounces yeast
6 cups lukewarm water
1 2/3 ounces maple syrup (if desired)

Mix together well, then knead for at least 10 minutes and let rise for another 10 minutes. Then add:

2/3 ounce sea salt
1 2/3 ounces cold-pressed vegetable oil

Knead until the dough is smooth. Form into small balls, roll in the black cumin seeds, and bake on the upper level of the oven at 250°C for about 20 – 25 minutes.

Indian Flat Bread (Chapatis)

Ingredients: 1/2 lb. fine whole-wheat or whole-rye flour
1/2 teaspoon finely ground black cumin seeds
1 teaspoon sea salt
Approx. 150 ml water

Mix the flour with the spices in a bowl. Gradually add the water and knead into the mixture until the dough is smooth. Let the dough rise for about 20 minutes. Roll out into thin flat breads (stated amount of flour is enough for about 6 pieces) and bake in an iron pan (for experts: directly on the stove plate) until golden brown on both sides.

Arabian Flat Bread (from the Oven)

Ingredients: 1 lb. fine whole-wheat flour
1 small package of yeast
Approx. 6 cups lukewarm water
1/2 cup cold-pressed oil
1/2 – 1 teaspoon salt
1/2 – 1 teaspoon finely ground black cumin
seeds
whole black cumin to sprinkle on bread

Knead the flour into a dough by adding the yeast with the water. Let rise for 15 minutes. Add oil, salt, and black cumin to it and knead once again. Roll out into flat breads the size of plates (given amount of flour is enough for about 4 pieces). Sprinkle with black cumin (and, if desired, with sesame), and bake on the upper level of the oven for about 10 minutes.

FINE SPICE PASTRIES

Ingredients: 1/2 lb. whole-wheat flour
1/2 small package of yeast
2 cups lukewarm water
1 teaspoon honey

Knead into a dough and let rise for 15 minutes. Then add:

2 2/3 ounces melted butter or margarine
2 2/3 ounces ground almonds or hazelnuts
2 ounces honey
Grated peel of 1/2 organically grown lemon
1 teaspoon cinnamon
1 teaspoon ground black cumin seeds
1 pinch of ginger, cloves, nutmeg

Knead in well and fill into a baking tin. Let rise for another 15 minutes. Bake in the oven at 200°C for about 1 hour.

... In closing, for the sake of better digestion here are a few:

Delicious Drinks

Power Drink à la Renate

Warm 1 large cup of milk, stir in 1 – 2 teaspoons of black cumin oil, and mix 1 teaspoon of mild honey of blossoms and flowers or maple syrup in well. As refinement: whipped-cream topping with grated chocolate.

❀ *We all need power for the long run ...*

Arabian Mocca

Put 1 pinch each of finely ground black cumin and cardamon into coffee; it must be a dark roasted Arabica variety, at best true Jemenite mocca. If you grind your own coffee beans, you can put the seeds into the mill in a ratio of 6:1.

❀ *Wonderful after a feast ...*

Nigellina Tea "Fragrance of the Orient"

Pour 1 large cup of water that is almost boiling over 1 table-spoon of finely ground black cumin seeds. Let draw for 8 – 10 minutes. Flavor with milk or cream, honey, and 1 pinch of vanilla.

❀ *Gives us sweet dreams in a 1001 Nights ...*

APPENDIX

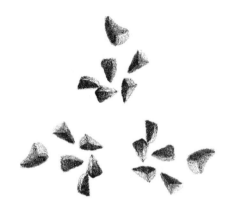

Analyzes Results

PRODUCT: BLACK CUMIN OIL
Carefully cold-pressed with protection against oxidation

ÖHMI Test No.:   L97.249.1
Analysis Date: June 9, 1997

Indicator	Dimension	Method	Black Cumin Oil
Peroxide value	mval/kg	DGF C-VI 6a	13.0 x
Free fatty acids	%	DGF C-III 4	2.80
Saponifiable	%	DGF C-III 1a	76.2

Composition of Fatty Acids:

Myristic acid	C14	–
Palmitic acid	C16	13.90
Palmitoleic acid	C16:1	0.18
Heptadecanoic acid	C17	–
Heptadecaenoic acid	C17:1	–
Stearic acid	C18	2.69
Oleic acid	C18:1	23.63
Linoleic acid	C18:2	56.87
Linolenic acid	C18:3a	0.14
Linolenic acid	C18:3y	–
Stearidonic acid	C18:4	–
Arachidic acid	C20	0.11
Eicosaenic acid	C20:1	0.18
	C20:2	1.98
Behenic acid	C22	0.04
Erucic acid	C22:1	–
Lignocerinic acid	C24	–
Traces	–	

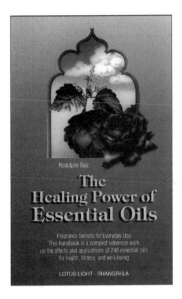

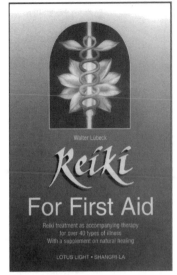

Rodolphe Balz

**The Healing Power
of Essential Oils**

**Fragrance Secrets for Everyday
Use. This handbook is a compact
reference work on the effects and
applications of 248 essential oils
for health, fitness, and well-being**

Fifteen years of organic cultivation of
spice plants and healing herbs in the
French Provence have provided
Rodolphe Balz with extensive knowledge about essential oils, how they
work, and how to use them.
The heart of *The Healing Power of
Essential Oils* is an essenial-oil index
describing their properties, followed
by a comprehensive therapeutic index for putting them to practical use.
Further topics of this indispensible
aromatherapy handbook are distillation processes, concentrations,
chemotypes, quality and quality control, toxicity, self-medication, and the
aromatogram.

208 pages, $ 14.95
ISBN 0-941524-89-2

Walter Lübeck

Reiki For First Aid

**Reiki Treatment as Accompanying
Therapy for over 40 Types
of Illness
With a Supplement on
Natural Healing**

Reiki For First Aid offers much practical advice for applying the universal life force in everyday health care.
The book includes Reiki treatments
for over forty types of illness, supplemented with natural-healing applications and a detailed description of
the relationship between Reiki and
nutrition.
Reiki Master Walter Lübeck gives
extensive instructions on topics rang-
ing from Reiki whole-body treatments to special positions. These
special Reiki treatment positions are
an important contribution to the field
of natural healing.

160 pages, $ 14.95
ISBN 0-914955-26-8

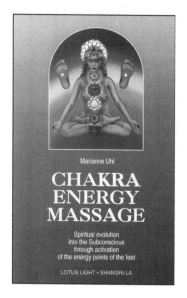

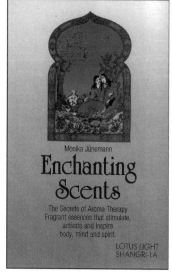

Marianne Uhl

Chakra Energy Massage

Spiritual Evolution in the Subconscious by Activating of the Energy Points of the Feet

This book guides you into the fascinating world of the energy body. Based on the knowledge of foot reflexology massage it introduces you to chakra energy massage, which can activate the individual energy centers of the human body. By means of the fine energy channels connecting them to the body's organs and energy centers, the feet reflect our physical and psychological condition. The author enables you to quickly acquire all of the knowledge needed for foot reflexology massage and chakra energy massage. In addition, she provides information on the vibrations of primal tones and various colors to effectively enhance your work with the chakras.

128 pages, $ 9.95
ISBN 0-941524-83-3

Monika Jünemann

Enchanting Scents

The Secrets of Aromatherapy Fragrant Essences that Stimulate, Activate and Inspire Body, Mind and Spirit

Today we are just as captivated by the magic of lovely scents and as irresistably moved by them as ever. The effects that essential oils have can vary greatly. This book particularly treats their subtle influences, but also presents and describes the plants from which they are obtained. It beckons you to enter the realm of sensual experience and journey into the world of fragrance through essences. It is an invitation to use personal scents to activate body and spirit. Here is a key that will open your senses to the limitless possibilities of benefitting from fragrances as stimulants, sources of energy, and means of healing.

128 pages, $ 9. 95
ISBN 0-941524-36-1

Planetary Herbology

CD Version / Win 95

The Planetary Herbology software program is the perfect companion to the book *Planetary Herbology* by Dr. Michael Tierra, one of the best-known herbalists in the world. The program unifies planetary approaches to ⁓rbal health, including Chinese, Western, Ayurvedic and ⁓ve American herbal wisdom.

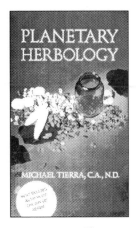

⁓ompletely updated and expanded version of the ⁓laimed planetary herbology computer program, this ⁓ ROM comes with the complete program developed ⁓r use under Windows 95. It contains 134 color photos ⁓f herbs. The research editor comes with and fully ⁓ntegrates into the program allowing you to add your own comments and information to the files. There is a context-sensitive help file. The program features extremely powerful intuitive and boolean search abilities. It allows you to print to a file or to a printer. In all, 464 herbs and formulas are covered. Over 3700 listings make sense of the conditions and symptoms. Over 3000 listings detail the action of herbs. You can search by herb common name, herb Latin name, condition or symptom, actions and properties of the herbs, and constituents of the herbs. Definitions of all herbal properties and many constituents of herbs are included at the click of a mouse.

System Requirements: IBM compatible running under Windows 95. CD ROM required for installation. Minimum 486 class 66 mhz. 16 MB RAM. Requires 40 MB hard disk space for installation. Mouse and color monitor required.

Dos/Win 3.1 USERS: If you are running DOS or Windows 3.1 you can still get the benefit of this extraordinary program by ordering our original *Planetary Herbology* Software for DOS/Win 3.1. Note that the Dos/Win 3.1 version is on 3.5 or 5 1/4" floppy disk and that the research editor for that version is sold separately. The Dos/Win 3.1 version requires 512K of RAM and 8 MB of hard disk space to be installed and operate. While this version will also function under Windows 95, it will not have the enhanced capabilities of the Win / 95 version, for instance the color photos.

ORDERING AND FURTHER INFORMATION:
Both versions are available either together with the book *Planetary Herbology* by Michael Tierra or ordered separately. Ask your local bookseller or natural foods store or contact us directly:

990124	Planetary Herbology (book), Michael Tierra	ISBN 0 941524-27-2	490 pp	$17.95
990107	Planetary Herbology Book with Windows 95 Program CD: includes Research Editor and Color Photos free			$69.95
990108	Planetary Herbology Windows 95 Program CD (without book): includes Research Editor and Color Photos free			$59.95
990102	Planetary Herbology Book with DOS/Win 3.1 Program Disks:			$65.00
990103	Planetary Herbology DOS/Win 3.1 Program Disks (without book):			$55.00
990104	Planetary Herbology Research Editor Upgrade for DOS/Win 3.1 version:			$50.00

Lotus Press, PO Box 325   Twin Lakes, WI 53181. 800 824 6396 (order line);
414 889 8561 (office phone); 414 889 8591 (fax line);
email: lotuspress@lotuspress.com   web site: www.lotuspress.com

Sources of Supply:

The following companies have an extensive selection of useful products and a long track-record of fulfillment. They have natural body care, aromatherapy, flower essences, crystals and tumbled stones, homeopathy, herbal products, vitamins and supplements, videos, books, audio tapes, candles, incense and bulk herbs, teas, massage tools and products and numerous alternative health items across a wide range of categories.

WHOLESALE:

Wholesale suppliers sell to stores and practitioners, not to individual consumers buying for their own personal use. Individual consumers should contact the RETAIL supplier listed below. Wholesale accounts should contact with business name, resale number or practitioner license in order to obtain a wholesale catalog and set up an account.

Lotus Light Enterprises, Inc.

P O Box 1008 BC
Silver Lake, WI 53170 USA
414 889 8501 (phone)
414 889 8591 (fax)
800 548 3824 (toll free order line)

RETAIL:

Retail suppliers provide products by mail order direct to consumers for their personal use. Stores or practitioners should contact the wholesale supplier listed above.

Internatural

33719 116th Street BC
Twin Lakes, WI 53181 USA
800 643 4221 (toll free order line)
414 889 8581 office phone
WEB SITE: www.internatural.com

Web site includes an extensive annotated catalog of more than 7000 products that can be ordered "on line" for your convenience 24 hours a day, 7 days a week.